Inducing Immunity?

Basic Bioethics

Art Caplan, editor

A complete list of the books in the Basic Bioethics series appears at the back of this book.

Inducing Immunity?

Justifying Immunization Policies in Times of Vaccine Hesitancy

Roland Pierik and Marcel Verweij

The MIT Press
Cambridge, Massachusetts
London, England

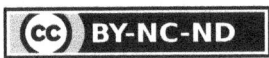
TThe MIT Press would like to thank the anonymous peer reviewers who provided comments on drafts of this book. The generous work of academic experts is essential for establishing the authority and quality of our publications. We acknowledge with gratitude the contributions of these otherwise uncredited readers.

This book was set in Stone Serif and Stone Sans by Westchester Publishing Services. Printed and bound in the United States of America.

Library of Congress Cataloging-in-Publication Data

Names: Pierik, Roland H. M., author. | Verweij, M. F., author.
Title: Inducing immunity? : justifying immunization policies in times of vaccine hesitancy / Roland Pierik and Marcel Verweij.
Other titles: Basic bioethics
Description: Cambridge, Massachusetts : The MIT Press, [2024] | Series: Basic bioethics | Includes bibliographical references and index.
Identifiers: LCCN 2023013919 (print) | LCCN 2023013920 (ebook) | ISBN 9780262547796 (paperback) | ISBN 9780262378369 (epub) | ISBN 9780262378376 (PDF)
Subjects: MESH: Vaccination—ethics | Mandatory Programs—ethics | Vaccination Hesitancy | Health Policy | Communicable Disease Control
Classification: LCC RA638 (print) | LCC RA638 (ebook) | NLM WA 115 | DDC 614.4/7—dc23/eng/20230727
LC record available at https://lccn.loc.gov/2023013919
LC ebook record available at https://lccn.loc.gov/2023013920

10 9 8 7 6 5 4 3 2

Contents

Preface

The work on this book has taken much longer than we could have imagined when we started the project. The first trigger for thinking about an in-depth ethical and legal analysis of immunization policies was the 2013–2014 measles outbreak in the Netherlands, which primarily affected religious communities with low vaccine coverage. Reported cases of measles stood at 2700, 182 children were hospitalized, and one child died from complications. This outbreak could be seen as just another in a long series of measles and poliomyelitis outbreaks in the Bible Belt in The Netherlands, where members of orthodox reformed churches live together in close-knit communities and often refuse vaccination for their children. We were intrigued by the lukewarm reaction of politicians and policymakers to the impact of this outbreak. Prime Minister Mark Rutte went no further than merely recommending that parents get their children vaccinated. The general political stance was that—hopefully—vaccination rates would increase through persuasion and education. Mandatory vaccination was considered to be futile because objectors would not comply anyway. We were surprised by these restrained reactions. Why were such outbreaks and the vaccine refusal of these parents perceived as immutable facts of life? And why were more coercive vaccination policies not even considered as ways to protect children against these diseases?

Religious objections have ceased to be the only grounds for vaccine hesitance and refusal. Since the turn of the millennium, new forms of vaccine hesitancy have emerged in many parts of the world, fueled by an increasingly vocal antivaccination movement. Supporters of this movement promulgate the idea that the dangers of vaccination far outweigh its benefit and seek to carve out "all-natural" lives for themselves and their children. At the same time, they tap into and reinforce an increasing lack of trust in vaccination programs, the medical establishment, and the state. This has resulted in an increased number of pockets of under-vaccination in many countries, and ultimately led to outbreaks of vaccine-preventable diseases. The infamous 2015 Disneyland outbreak in California made it abundantly clear that vaccine hesitancy could bring back diseases that (at least in high-income countries) had been safely under control for decades. In 2019, the World Health Organization (WHO) identified vaccine hesitancy as among the top health threats. It is remarkable that this health threat is not caused by a lack of a medical treatment for a serious disease: on the contrary, vaccines that are proven to be safe and effective are, at least in high-income countries, abundantly available. This health threat is caused by vaccine-hesitant persons' lack of trust in vaccines.

Looking at these events from a mindset that is informed by the COVID-19 pandemic, the mortality and morbidity of these outbreaks may seem limited. Yet even these "mild" epidemics of vaccine-preventable diseases touch a sensitive nerve in public debates and generate much political controversy. They confront liberal democracies with a difficult and morally-laden question: how should the state respond to citizens who refuse to participate in collective immunization programs that are meant to protect society at large and the health of children aged 16 or younger in particular? Should the government take a stronger stance by motivating, pressuring, or even compelling parents to accept vaccination?

Similar questions have emerged during the COVID-19 pandemic: should governments require adult citizens to have themselves and their children vaccinated, to prevent spread of infections, and counteract the societal disruption caused by the pandemic? Given that basic liberties and freedoms are at stake, such fundamental questions must be asked and answered, not only during a pandemic but also at times when vaccine-preventable disease are more or less under control.

This issue fitted well with our different research areas and expertise. Roland has extensive experience of analyzing the legal regulation of conflicting fundamental rights in liberal democracies and had just published a paper that takes a strong stance in favor of compulsory vaccination. Marcel has been working on the ethics of prevention and public health for decades and was deeply involved in policy advice work for the Health Council of the Netherlands. So, we decided to embark on a joint project: to analyze in depth the problem of how to regulate collective vaccination for children and adults in times of vaccine hesitance.

From the very beginning, the project concerned more than a topic of mere academic interest. The Disney measles outbreak and a series of measles outbreaks in Europe made several states and countries implement more coercive childhood vaccination policies, leaving parents less freedom to opt out (Navin & Attwell, 2023). Governments, professionals, and public and private organizations put more emphasis on countervailing misinformation about vaccination. This was all highly controversial and public debates on this issue became more and more tense and polarized.

And then the COVID-19 pandemic emerged, which necessitated drastic public health measures. This triggered even more debate, especially when vaccines became available and governments rolled out mass immunization campaigns. We became heavily involved in these societal debates and in policy advisory roles. This inevitably slowed down the work on our book manuscript, but it also helped to test, apply, and improve our analyses. In the meantime, Roland joined the temporary committee on medical aspects of COVID-19 of Health Council of the Netherlands. Many of the proposals and arguments in this book have emerged from, and have been further elucidated through insights from our advisory work for parliament, ministries, and public health agencies. Arguments were often initially developed in op-ed articles we published in national newspapers.

Our role in public debate thus delayed the progress of the book project but also improved the quality of the argument. In our experience, doing work on legal and political philosophy is much more relevant, fruitful, and interesting if it interacts with, and actually contributes to policy making and public deliberation. Our discussions with practitioners in the field and political decision makers provided us with a wealth of situational knowledge. Political philosophy and ethics helped us to outline, test and justify practical proposals; taking contextual factors and the complexities of public health practice into account also enabled us to adjust and further develop theoretical and principled arguments in moral and political philosophy.

This book therefore combines philosophical analysis with practical policy proposals, and this combination recognizes the importance of fundamental individual rights, the role of democratic decision making, and the inherent tension between the two. Ultimately, however, the question about how the state should respond to vaccine hesitance cannot be decided by ethical analysis alone. An ethically justified approach to vaccination can only become legitimate when it is discussed in public debates and is ultimately the outcome of a democratic process in which all relevant interests have been taken into account, especially the special protection that fundamental rights deserve. The fact that this is such a controversial topic only reinforces the importance of such a democratic process.

The controversy surrounding this theme was both a blessing and burden. On the one hand, we enjoyed having our op-eds published and being able to discuss our ideas on national radio and TV. It is a godsend for an academic if their research topic suddenly becomes world news. On the other hand, we also experienced personally how polarized the societal debate had become; there were disagreements not only on the status of normative principles and fundamental liberties but also, increasingly, about which facts, institutions, and people can be trusted and which cannot. In such a context, it will often be impossible to develop a discussion merely by offering a philosophical analysis. The angry responses, insults, and personal threats we received made it clear that some citizens considered us to be dangerous, self-interested, untrustworthy nonexperts who were probably paid by the pharmaceutical industry or government to prepare society for a new world order.

These extreme reactions may be characteristic of societal debates nowadays. At the same time, we see that most policy makers, politicians, scientists, and co-citizens are very interested in, and open to philosophical reflection on the dilemmas that arise in times of vaccine hesitance. The fact that public debate is sometimes overheated does not imply that we should abandon critical ethical reflection on a topic like this. Ideally our book will contribute to fundamental debates in philosophy of law and ethics, but especially also to political decision making and responsible vaccination policies. We hope that it will not only be read and discussed in academic circles, but also by professionals and policymakers in public health. Even though a large part of our analysis centers around the idea of proportionality, which is most prominent in the European legal tradition, the overall argument is relevant in any liberal democratic jurisdiction, including the United States of America.

While we were writing this book, many academics and practitioners in the field engaged with our project. We have learned a lot from discussions with scientists in the Health Council of the Netherlands (Gezondheidsraad) and from our various interactions with infectious disease specialists from the

National Institute for Public Health and the Environment (RIVM) and the WHO. It was great to discuss some early chapters with our colleagues at the Philosophy chair group at Wageningen University and the Paul Scholten Centre for Jurisprudence at the University of Amsterdam. We are especially grateful for the generous comments we received at a manuscript symposium in October 2021 in Amsterdam. Justin Bernstein, Alberto Giubilini, Mariëtte van den Hoven, Steven Kraaijeveld, Mark Navin, Dorit Reiss, and Brigit Toebes had read the first complete draft and offered in-depth critical yet constructive feedback. We also want to thank the reviewers for their suggestions that helped us to improve many small and larger arguments in the book. Parts of the book build on analyses we have published in papers in academic journals, including *Public Health Ethics*, *Vaccine*, *Journal of Applied Philosophy*, *Ethnicities*, *American Journal of Bioethics*, *het Tijdschrift voor Recht en Religie*, and *het Nederlands Juristenblad*. Section 4.4 is more or less a reprint of Marcel's paper "The (un)fairness of vaccination free riding," published in *Public Health Ethics*. We are grateful for being able to use this earlier work.

The societal debates, epidemiological developments, and all the academic interactions and contributions to policy making may have significantly delayed the completion of the book. At the same time, all these interactions made this project an endeavor that we enjoyed immensely. They have been invaluable in the development of the central line of our argument and our discussion of policy options for regulating collective immunization. We are grateful for all these opportunities, and we genuinely want to thank everyone who directly or indirectly contributed to this work. We also express our gratitude for the financial support we received from the Netherlands Organization for Health Research and Development (ZonMW 522004004).

May 2023

Marcel Verweij and Roland Pierik

1 Controversies and Complexities of Vaccination: An Introduction

Since Edward Jenner's first tests inoculating people with a cowpox-infected substance to protect them against smallpox at the end of the eighteenth century, and the immunization movements and policies that developed rapidly afterward, vaccination has become simultaneously a lauded and a controversial phenomenon. It has been highly successful in reducing outbreaks of infectious diseases and has been embraced by a large majority of populations in all countries, but at the same time, it has always been met with criticism, doubt, and resistance. Coverage of vaccines that protect against diseases such as diphtheria, tetanus, polio, pertussis, and measles is high in high-income countries, as well as in many middle- and low-income countries. Vaccination has led to the global eradication of smallpox and to the elimination of polio in almost all regions worldwide. Measles and other diseases that only decades ago were still considered inevitable and potentially dangerous childhood diseases are now relatively rare, at least in affluent countries.

Not all citizens take the benefits of immunization for granted, however: some people question the necessity of vaccination, claim that the risks of vaccination outweigh the benefits, or argue that preventive vaccination conflicts with their religious or secular worldviews. People thus appeal to a variety of concerns to forgo or resist vaccination for themselves or their children. Even countries with a high immunization coverage usually face local pockets of undervaccination (e.g., religious communities in the US and the Netherlands) in which outbreaks of vaccine-preventable diseases remain a constant threat. Moreover, the same general doubts about immunization complicate proposals for introducing novel vaccines and vaccination programs, like in the recent COVID-19 pandemic. We start this chapter with three examples that illustrate these concerns: the reemergence of measles outbreaks due to declining immunization rates, the low uptake of the relatively new vaccine against human papillomavirus, and deep controversies about immunization during the COVID-19 pandemic. The three cases set the stage for our analysis of the central problem in this book: what policies can be ethically, legally, and politically justified in response to vaccine hesitancy?

1.1   The 2014 Measles Outbreak in the US

Measles is one of the most contagious infectious diseases. An unvaccinated person who is exposed to the virus has a 90 percent chance of becoming infected. The disease kills one person in every 5,000 cases in high-income countries and as many as one person in every 100 cases in low-income countries (Oxford Vaccine Group, 2015). The risk of serious complications and death is increased in children younger than five years and adults older than twenty years (Strebel, 2018). On a global scale, measles kills 135,000 persons each year, mostly children (World Health Organization, 2019). In the 1960s, a live-attenuated measles vaccine was introduced for children aged around fourteen months. A decade later, this vaccine was included in the MMR (measles, mumps, rubella) triple vaccine, which is mostly given to children at around the age of fourteen months and again at nine years old. Vaccination has contributed to a stark reduction in measles cases in many regions, but outbreaks are still observed in regions with clusters of under-vaccination, such as the Bible Belt in the Netherlands. In 2000, the disease was declared eliminated in the US (Nigel et al., 2004). Since then, however, new outbreaks have occurred there. Among the twenty-three outbreaks in the US in 2014, there was one large outbreak, 383 cases, that occurred primarily among unvaccinated Amish communities in Ohio (Sundaram et al., 2019). Early in 2015, a multistate outbreak occurred that originated from infections in Disneyland in California, causing illness in around 150 mostly unvaccinated persons, children as well as adults (Jalabi, 2015). Even though the number of outbreaks in 2015 was not dramatically higher than in earlier years, the Disneyland outbreak caught the attention of vaccinating parents who realized that the emerging vaccine hesitancy could bring back diseases that had been under control for decades (Hausman, 2019). The Disneyland outbreak thus focused both societal and political attention on the impact of vaccine hesitancy, vaccine refusers, and the antivaccination movement. Although childhood vaccinations are mandatory in all states in the US, more and more parents have been granted personal belief exemptions, facilitating new outbreaks such as the one in Disneyland. The controversy about such clusters of infectious diseases led to new state legislation (in California and in other states) tightening mandatory immunization programs or abandoning personal belief exemptions altogether (Navin & Attwell, 2023).

1.2   Unpopular from the Start: Vaccination against Human Papillomavirus

In 2006, a vaccine became available against human papillomavirus (HPV), and it was relatively quickly adopted over the next few years in many countries worldwide. HPV infections are the most important cause of cervical cancer, which causes around 270,000 deaths a year, mostly in low- and middle-income countries. Compared to existing vaccines, the HPV vaccine was relatively novel as the aim was not so much to protect against HPV as a symptomatic infectious disease but against the harmful effects of sustained infection over time. Two other novelties were the fact that HPV is first and foremost a sexually transmittable infection and that the main target group for vaccination was, at that time, girls who were not yet sexually active. These aspects and concerns about alleged side effects featured in public debate, and at least in some countries, such as the Netherlands, the initial vaccine coverage was much lower than envisaged (Gefenaite et al., 2012). The Dutch program was initiated in 2009, targeting eleven- and twelve-year-old girls and including a one-off catchup program for thirteen- to sixteen-year-old girls. In the first few years, immunization coverage barely exceeded 50 percent, which was much lower than the 95 percent vaccination rates that were normally realized in infant immunization schemes in the Netherlands (van Lier et al., 2011). For the first time, governments were confronted with a massive public debate on social media featuring hesitance about and active resistance toward vaccination, showing distrust in health authorities, and highlighting rumors and fears.

1.3   Polarization in the COVID-19 Pandemic

The COVID-19 pandemic that began in 2020 and was caused by the SARS-CoV-2 virus has made it patently clear that massive epidemics are not phenomena that only affected a distant past—they can still acutely disrupt current societies. In many places in the world, dramatic societal measures were imposed to control infection rates, to protect the health and save the lives of citizens, and to sustain health care facilities that were overwhelmed by the influx of seriously ill patients. Around half of the world's populations faced national lockdowns that included travel restrictions and the closure of schools, universities, shops, and other businesses, and people were often expected, and sometimes forced, to stay at home as much as possible. Large public and private investments in vaccine development resulted in the development, approval, and mass production of vaccines in less than a year, and those vaccines appeared to be highly effective. Mass vaccination was generally considered the most important strategy for containing the pandemic and abandoning or relaxing lockdown measures, but many people also had doubts about the safety of these novel vaccines. Vaccine hesitancy and refusal were reinforced by misinformation: it was claimed that the vaccines resulted in many adverse events, and the pandemic itself was considered a lie made up by governments that just wanted to control citizens. It was also suggested that vaccines would modify people's genetic makeup or that they contained microchips that enabled governments to track citizens. Not all vaccine hesitancy, however, should be directly linked to (some of the more outrageous forms of) fake news. For example, given the speed of vaccine development, it should not have been a surprise that people had concerns about safety. Regardless of the background of hesitancy in different societies, debates about vaccination became more and more polarized during the later waves of the pandemic, especially when health care systems and intensive care units were flooded and sometimes overwhelmed with mostly unvaccinated patients.

In contrast to other vaccination-related controversies, this time it was not so much about childhood immunization but about the vaccination of adults, who, unlike children, are considered to have a far-reaching authority to make their own choices about medical treatments. Yet the context of a global pandemic, with dramatic infection control measures already in place, gave governments a very broad palette of policy opportunities, including more coercive approaches, to persuade or force citizens to get vaccinated. For example, some citizens were required to show so-called COVID-19 admission passes (cf. section 8.3) to access social events, pubs, and restaurants and, in some cases, even to be allowed into their workplace. All these discussions led to further polarization and division between citizens who embraced the immunization program, including subsequent boosters, and those who refused COVID-19 vaccines.

1.4   Vaccination Policies in Times of Resistance: An Uphill Battle?

Public health authorities are struggling with questions concerning how to respond to a lack of confidence in or even public distrust of vaccines and vaccination programs and how to shape policies that ensure the protection of public health. The controversies about vaccine hesitancy in the preceding sections (measles, HPV, and COVID-19) illustrate some of the key complexities that surround immunization policies.

One complexity is that vaccination involves individual choices that have public consequences and vice versa. The COVID-19 pandemic has shown how polarized debates can reinforce vaccine hesitance and refusal, which in turn impede societal attempts to overcome the pandemic. In relation to measles and other childhood diseases, many vaccine-hesitant parents assume that the benefits of vaccinations for their child, or for society in general, do not outweigh the risks they associate with vaccination. Yet their choice to forgo immunization not only affects the interests of their own child but also contributes to a decreased level of protection on a group level, which creates increased risk for those who cannot be vaccinated, for example, children who are too young to receive their first shot or (vaccinated) persons whose immune systems are weakened due to disease or other conditions. For various reasons, these aspects are less prominent in relation to HPV vaccination, but HPV did show how a public immunization policy has implications for issues that are considered rather personal and private matters: preadolescent girls and their parents were forced to think about sexual activity and the risk of acquiring sexually transmitted infections. For many parents and girls, this is a sensitive topic that they might prefer to avoid discussing.

A second complexity of immunization programs is that they aim to *prevent* disease, so their success is often a remote, if not invisible, entity to individuals. This may not be the case during an epidemic, but it is certainly so for most routine (childhood) vaccination programs. In normal circumstances, programs are implemented when there is no threat of an acute outbreak. Teenagers are vaccinated against HPV to protect them against a disease in the distant future. As humans, we consider ourselves rational beings, but we can easily neglect or discount long-term risks. Moreover, our knowledge of the benefits of vaccination is often distorted because its success is only visible on a population level. For individual persons, the effect of a successful vaccination is a nonevent: they are not infected and thus remain healthy. Yet no one will ever know whether they would have become ill if they had not been vaccinated. This complexity makes it more difficult to persuade people by pointing out the benefit of immunization. And vaccination failure—cases of infection that occur notwithstanding the fact that the person was vaccinated—always stands out, and so do (alleged) side effects of vaccinations. Hence, it is no surprise that public health authorities and medical professionals sometimes struggle to persuade hesitant parents to accept immunization of their children. A full assessment of the benefits and burdens cannot be made by appealing to individual observations but requires a population perspective—that is, an evaluation of the epidemiological evidence concerning infection risks and vaccination safety.

This also brings a third complexity and controversy to the surface. Vaccination programs should be based on robust scientific evidence about infection risks and vaccine effectiveness and safety. Ideally, such evidence also helps to persuade citizens to endorse immunization and participate in programs. Most people, however, do not make up their mind on the basis of a rational assessment of the available evidence. They often defer to expert assessment or simply trust their general practitioner or other health care professionals. But choices are also affected by experiences with previous vaccinations, personal anecdotes of friends, and stories shared on social media—and these can easily exaggerate concerns about safety and downplay the importance of immunization. Nowadays, people are confronted with an abundance of information and perspectives via the internet and other media—including some sources that are reliable and others that are not. Moreover, a lot of deliberate misinformation and messages are available that aim to trigger doubt and skepticism about vaccines (Donzelli et al., 2018; Ginossar et al., 2022; Wolfe et al., 2023). Governments cannot and should not assume that the provision of good, reliable information will guarantee a high uptake in collective immunization programs. Such (often abstract) information is certainly necessary, but it will also be rather ineffective in persuading citizens who are already skeptical about experts or governments.

The diversity of the vaccine-hesitant population (cf. chapter 3) constitutes a fourth complexity for public health programs. Given the—often invisible—benefits of immunization, it is not strange that many people pay more attention to possible side effects and therefore postpone or forgo immunization. Yet it is not just the alleged side effects of immunization that lead people to avoid vaccines. Several religious groups consider immunization (or some forms of disease prevention in general) to be an act that seeks to preempt divine providence. If parents assume that the health of their children is in the hands of God, they may conclude that it is not up to them to prevent illness by means of immunization. Nonreligious worldviews can also motivate vaccine hesitance, for example, a view that emphasizes "naturalness," "purity," or the innocence of infants—suggesting that vaccination interferes in natural processes that are good in themselves. Anthroposophist groups see "childhood diseases" as important stages in childhood development and consider coming through such an illness as ultimately beneficial for the child. Finally, some groups reject vaccination programs for more political reasons. If one sees any government policy as intruding in the private lives of citizens, then it may easily follow that government-imposed collective immunization programs are evil. These diverse motives for vaccine hesitance can also reinforce one other, and different groups may find each other when fighting for a similar objective: to resist government-led immunization programs.

The complexities surrounding collective vaccination pose a deep problem for public health authorities and governments. High immunization rates are necessary to protect against potentially dangerous diseases. Vaccine hesitancy may well result in a comeback of almost forgotten diseases such as measles, diphtheria, or polio, and it inhibits effective government responses to pandemics or other disease outbreaks. But if, given the complexities just mentioned, it is not to be expected that evidence-based information will persuade vaccine-hesitant persons to get vaccinated, the question arises what public health authorities should do. To what extent should citizens with doubts about immunization or those who actively resist it be persuaded, pressured, or legally obliged to accept it? What is the role of government in this controversy? These are the main questions that we will explore in this book. Before outlining our approach, let us first look in more detail at what vaccination is and how collective immunization programs have evolved throughout the centuries.

1.5 Immunization and Immunization Programs

Vaccines have become one of the most important tools of preventive medicine against certain virus- and bacteria-induced diseases. For infections with viruses, there is often no curative therapy; they can only be countered by an organism's immune system. Vaccination is the deliberate exposure of an organism to a weakened or killed version of a pathogenic microbe, or just a part of that pathogen, to induce the organism to produce antibodies. This initial production of vaccine-specific antibodies enables the immune system to recognize a "real" pathogen if exposed to it and to rapidly produce antibodies to fight it. Hence, a successful vaccine triggers the immune system and thus "immunizes" the organism against the pathogen, without inducing the actual disease and the risks it generates. Throughout the book, we will use the terms "immunization" and "vaccination" as synonyms, although, strictly speaking, "immunization" also includes other ways to induce immunity—such as via "real" infections or inoculation.

Long before Edward Jenner started experimenting with *variola vaccinae*, or cowpox, as a way to protect humans against *variola*, or smallpox, it was common in some societies to inoculate persons with smallpox pus or scabs, either by inserting some pus from a patient with smallpox into an incision in the skin of another person or by blowing powdered scabs into a person's nostrils. In China, the practice of inoculation, or *variolation*, was described as early as the eleventh century, but it probably started in India, perhaps before the Christian era (Hopkins, 2002, p. 109). One description of early inoculation can be found in *Zhou Hou Bei Ji Fan* by Ge Hong (283–363), published around AD 303. Ge Hong describes a form of preventive exposure to rabies: "killing the dog that bites, and using its brain for the people who will be safe without relapse of rabies" (Cao, 2008). Presumably, the risks of such inoculations themselves causing and spreading the disease were significant.

Smallpox inoculation was introduced in Western Europe early in the eighteenth century and was enthusiastically practiced by several physicians throughout the century, including the Gloucestershire physician and scientist Edward Jenner. Jenner started studying cowpox that developed on the hands of milkmaids; he was fascinated by stories about milkmaids who had been infected with cowpox—a rather innocent condition in cattle—but remained healthy when they were exposed to smallpox at a later date. His first experiments, however, involved swine pox. Jenner did tests on several persons, including his own son, exposing them via an incision to swine pox pus and later on inoculating them with smallpox. On May 14, 1796, he carried out the famous experiment on James Phipps, the eight-year-old son of his gardener. Jenner first inoculated the boy with pus from the blisters of Sarah Nelms, a Gloucestershire milkmaid who had recently been infected with cowpox. One and a half months later, James Phipps was inoculated again, this time with pus from a patient with smallpox. This caused only a mild infection. Edward Jenner's first scientific report was not well received by the British Royal Society—the opinion was that if he valued his reputation, he would have been better not promulgating such ideas. But after he had done more experiments and published them in his *Inquiry*, the idea of *variolation vaccinae* swiftly became more accepted—although never without controversy. Within three years after its English publication, the *Inquiry* was translated into French, Dutch, Spanish, Russian, Italian, and Latin. Jenner and many others strongly promoted vaccination, and by the beginning of the nineteenth century, the procedure was carried out regularly in many European countries. By 1801, more than 100,000 persons had been vaccinated in Great Britain, and in the decade afterward, several million vaccinations were administered in countries such as Russia and France (Hopkins, 2002, p. 81).

It took almost a century before other vaccines became available. Louis Pasteur developed the idea that a virulent pathogen could be attenuated (i.e., weakened), most famously with his rabies vaccine, paving the way for a series of live-attenuated vaccines like yellow fever, polio, and measles in the twentieth century. Other vaccines were based upon killed pathogens, including cholera, the inactivated polio vaccine, and hepatitis A. From the last part of the twentieth century onward, a variety of novel vaccine technologies were developed. These include subunit vaccines that contain only a specific protein of the pathogen, such as pneumococcal, hepatitis B, and HPV vaccines. In the twenty-first century, viral vector and messenger RNA (mRNA) technologies were developed, which have been especially employed in several COVID-19 vaccines (Gergen & Petsch, 2020; Plotkin, 2014, p. 12284).

From the 1950s, government-led national immunization programs became more and more common, combining different vaccines and having a clear impact on outbreaks of diseases such as polio and measles. However, it is difficult to quantify the effects of collective vaccination, given that morbidity and mortality due to contagious diseases were already declining throughout the twentieth century (van Wijhe et al., 2016). Infectious diseases thrive in unhygienic conditions, poor households, and undernourished populations, so the improvement of hygiene and living conditions that came with increased economic prosperity in Western countries was already resulting in a steep decline of major infectious diseases. Good living conditions alone, however, will not rule out infections altogether, and children and adults—especially those who are relatively vulnerable—may still become seriously ill with infections that cause only mild disease in many others. Even healthy children are vulnerable to infections like measles, polio, and pertussis, and unless many individuals are immune, a contagious microbe can still spread rapidly within a population.

1.6 Vaccination Strategies

We can distinguish three major objectives for collective immunization. The most effective aim is the elimination or eradication of a serious infectious disease. The elimination of an infection implies the exclusion of the disease from a defined region, but a risk would still remain of reintroduction from another region. Eradication is the total exclusion of the relevant pathogen from the environment, so it cannot return. Less than 200 years after Edward Jenner's experiments, the global struggle against smallpox came to an end. The last victim of endemic smallpox was a Somalian boy in 1977.[1] In 1980, the World Health Organization declared that this disease, which scars those who have it and can often be fatal, had been eradicated globally, which also implied that the last remaining smallpox vaccination programs could be discontinued. The complete eradication of a dangerous disease offers not only perfect protection but also the opportunity to discontinue a specific vaccination, not only immediately but in the future. However, it is extremely hard to achieve this goal, and smallpox will probably remain more of an exception than a general rule, given the epidemiological properties of many other vaccine-preventable diseases.[2]

The eradication of a contagious disease can only be attained if a large part of the (global) population is vaccinated. Mass vaccinations can inhibit and eventually stop the spread of infection by inducing immunity in a large part of the population. Individuals who are immune to an infection, after vaccination or as a result of a previous infection, cannot transmit the pathogen to other persons. If many persons in a collective are immune, this reduces the chance that persons who still are vulnerable will be exposed to infection: they are relatively safe within the "herd." It also implies that there are few possibilities for the pathogen to find an organism in which it can survive and reproduce. As a result, eventual outbreaks will fade out soon. A high vaccination rate can thus result in group-level protection, or *herd immunity*. If elimination of the disease is unfeasible, achieving group-level protection can still be a second objective that is attainable. With such protection, outbreaks will rarely occur, the disease will not gain a foothold in the population, and individuals who are not (yet) vaccinated or not immune for other reasons are well protected in the crowd. For example, measles is an extremely contagious disease, which implies that a patient is not only a victim of the disease but also a vector in its further spread. Even if a child experiences only relatively mild symptoms, they remain an infection risk to others. Vaccination protects individuals, but infants six to twelve months old are too young to be vaccinated, and therefore they depend on group-level protection. The higher the vaccination rate, the better these vulnerable children are protected as well.

Not all vaccination programs can achieve herd immunity or elimination of a disease, for example, because the pathogen might not be contagious or because there may be other (nonhuman) hosts in which the microbe can reproduce. In such cases, a third objective of collective vaccination programs is to offer individual protection to as many individuals as possible.

1.7   The Effectiveness of Vaccination Programs

The extent to which vaccines and vaccination programs can generate individual and collective protection against a particular infectious disease depends on various factors. The first factor is contagiousness: the more infectious a disease is, the harder it is to fight the disease via vaccination programs. The second factor is the extent to which the vaccine protects the individual vaccinee against the disease and, negatively, the extent to which this protection decreases over time. The third is the extent to which the vaccine provides sterilizing immunity (i.e., prevention of transmission of the wild-type pathogen to curb an outbreak) and, negatively, the extent to which this protection wanes over time. A vaccine does not have to provide full sterilizing immunity to curb an outbreak. The whooping cough

Box 1.1

Herd Immunity

The commonly used term "herd immunity" might be slightly misleading because "immunity" falsely suggests full protection against outbreaks of a disease (Fox et al., 1971; Jones & Helmreich, 2020). Moreover, it also seems to assume that there is a threshold—a proportion of the population who have attained immunity through infection or vaccination—at which this full collective protection is achieved. For example, it has been estimated that 92 to 94 percent of a population needs to be vaccinated in order to achieve herd immunity for measles (Orenstein et al., 2007, p. 1434). In the case of polio, the threshold is around 80 percent (Macmillan, 2021). In theory, it might be possible to calculate a herd immunity threshold based on R_0, the average number of persons who are infected by one infectious individual.

In practice, however, such thresholds are highly problematic due to population heterogeneity: a country with a very high vaccination coverage will often still have local areas where fewer persons are immune, for example, because such communities resist immunization. Moreover, high-risk persons may have a very high number of interactions, facilitating the spread of disease in the larger population. It is therefore not obvious that a theoretical national immunity threshold is sufficient for preventing outbreaks.

The term "herd immunity" also suggests that in the herd, no infections can occur at all, and if it is absent, the population is at risk—but this dichotomy is too simple. Even if an ideal threshold vaccine coverage (e.g., 94 percent in the case of measles) is not attained, the crowd can still offer a very high level of protection to vulnerable individuals. In this sense, herd immunity is not a threshold concept, although in policy making, it will be useful to aim at and ascertain specific minimum thresholds for vaccine coverage.

In this book, we often use the term "group-level protection" to refer to collective protection that arises as a result of many individuals having immunity against a disease. When we use the common term "herd immunity," it refers to a very high level of such collective protection—something that comes close to theoretical thresholds as indicated above.

vaccine, the rotavirus vaccine, and the inactivated polio vaccine do not provide full sterilizing immunity, but a vaccine does contribute to controlling an outbreak when the number of infections remains limited, and it helps to reduce hospitalizations by curbing the severity of individual cases of the disease (McKenna, 2021). The fourth and last factor is the percentage of the population that is immunized.

The infectiousness of a disease is a background factor that often can't be changed. The second and third factors, however, can be adjusted. The effectiveness of different vaccines varies regarding preventing disease or infection. The measles vaccine is extremely effective in protecting against both severe disease and the spread of infection, and these protective effects hardly decline at all over time. The flu vaccine, on the other hand, reduces the risk of illness by only 40 to 60 percent among the overall population,[3] and its effect wanes very quickly because every year, new strains of the virus emerge; hence, the target group usually needs to be revaccinated every year. The effectiveness of vaccinations can be improved by changing their composition or other pharmacological innovations. But in a collective program, it is also possible to increase collective protection by optimizing *who* is vaccinated. If a vaccine is offering a large degree of sterile immunity, it becomes possible to protect the most vulnerable groups, not (or not only) by vaccinating them but by immunizing all individuals who play the largest role in the spread of infection—even if the latter would run no risk of contracting a severe case of the disease themselves. This would amount to what some have coined "altruist vaccination" (Kraaijeveld, 2020).

Our argument in this book primarily addresses the fourth factor that determines the effectiveness of collective immunization: the vaccination rate. Herd immunity for many diseases can be achieved only through mass vaccination programs. As previously mentioned, the measles vaccine is very effective, but the disease is extremely contagious, and therefore herd protection requires a vaccine coverage of approximately 92 to 94 percent (Orenstein et al., 2007, p. 1434). COVID-19 also requires a high vaccination rate, but as the current vaccines offer only limited protection against infection and their effect wanes over time, a robust herd protection seems unattainable. Given that the four factors just described differ significantly for different vaccines and given that effectiveness is crucial for the regulation of vaccination policies, it is important to discuss regulation not merely in a general way. It is possible to develop a normative (ethical and legal) argument for vaccination policies, and this is what most of this book aims to do. Determining which specific policy is justified in which circumstances and for what vaccines and diseases requires taking many contextual features into account, which we will do in chapters 7 and 8 in particular.

1.8   Regulating Vaccination in Times of Distrust and Controversy

The eradication of smallpox is clearly one of the greatest achievements of collective vaccination programs, but this is still the only disease that has been eliminated on a global scale. Other dangerous infectious agents like polio and diphtheria have been eliminated in most regions but not everywhere, so there is still a risk of reintroduction in areas where vaccine coverage is not optimal.

Given the scientific evidence about the effectiveness and safety of vaccines used in basic programs, governments and (non)governmental health agencies have strong reasons to promote such vaccination programs, to strive for immunization rates that are as high as possible, and to aim for herd immunity where that is technically possible. Throughout the second half of the twentieth century, achieving optimum vaccination coverage appeared feasible—at least in most high-income countries. Large-scale programs gained momentum thanks to the discoveries of new vaccines such as those against polio, the novel possibilities of mass vaccine production, and the involvement of charities and other nongovernmental health organizations such as the March of Dimes in the US and the White-Yellow Cross and Green Cross in the Netherlands.

Before vaccines were introduced, epidemics and child mortality due to common infections were still very common, and nonlethal diseases could leave patients permanently disabled or disfigured. All this contributed to broad acceptance of vaccines and vaccine policies, once they arrived. This is not to say that controversy and doubts about vaccination faded away completely. Some religious groups have resisted vaccination from the start because they see immunization as disrespecting divine providence. Outbreaks of diseases such as polio are more likely to occur where people are living together in close, homogenic communities, as happened, for example, in the Netherlands in 1971 and 1992. Many other people question either the safety or the medical benefits of vaccines and therefore forgo immunizations, as we have illustrated with the cases at the beginning of this chapter.

In this book, we discuss the ethical and political-philosophical questions concerning how immunization programs should be regulated by government, given the fact that certain groups wholeheartedly and vocally reject vaccination and that many parents are at least hesitant about having their child or themselves vaccinated. The principled argumentation in this book is generic, but we focus primarily on childhood vaccination because most programs target children. In chapter 8, we shift the focus to immunization of adults, using COVID-19 as a controversial illustration.[4]

1.9 Basic Assumptions, Research Question, and Theoretical Approach

In this book, we presuppose a constitutional liberal-democratic government, usually abbreviated as "liberal democracy" or "democracy," which refers to a political regime that favors the protection of fundamental rights, democratic decision-making, and the rule of law. There are at least four foundational values underlying legislation and policy making in such regimes (Pierik & Werner, 2010, p. 2). The first characterization of liberal-democratic thought is *normative individualism*. All persons, both adults and young children, are taken to be "self-originating sources of valid claims" and, as such, the ultimate units of concern (Rawls, 1980, p. 543). Liberal-democratic thought differs in this respect from political theories that take, for example, the family or ethnic or religious communities as units of moral concern in and of themselves. Such aspects are only considered valuable instrumentally if they play a role in making an individual's life better. Second, liberal-democratic thought is characterized by a strong commitment to *personal autonomy*: individuals have a right to live their life in accordance with their idea of the good life and to be free from unjustified interferences in their personal sphere by others, including the state. Third, liberal-democratic thought recognizes the fact of *reasonable disagreement* among the different conceptions of the good in current plural societies and that the state should aim to be neutral toward the various (reasonable) conceptions of the good. The fourth and final characteristic is *statism*: liberal-democratic thought presupposes a central role for the state in promoting personal autonomy and state neutrality and in proposing policies that solve the inherent conflicts between those goals in pluralist societies.

Yet, as minimal and general as this description of liberal-democratic thought might be, it does offer a fruitful starting point for analyzing the responsibility of governments in relation to public health, including the responsibility of the state to prevent diseases through collective immunization programs. Given the possible disruptive effects of such diseases, the state has a compelling interest in preventing outbreaks. Indeed, although it remains contested within some circles whether the liberal-democratic state should promote individual health and health equity through collective institutions,[5] it is not disputed that it should *protect* society against major threats to public health (Verweij & Houweling, 2014). This implies that the state must guarantee a basic level of protection against infectious diseases that undermine or disrupt societal life and threaten people's options for shaping their lives as they see fit, individually and with others—as long as the cost of doing so does less to undermine or disrupt societal life than the diseases do. After all, the cure should not be worse than the disease.

The argument in this book addresses societies with well-functioning public health infrastructures. Vaccination programs are an essential element of such infrastructures, and most people endorse immunization as an indispensable protection against infectious diseases, for their children or themselves. At the same time, there has always been a minority that opposes vaccination and questions the evidence behind immunization. This opposition becomes problematic when, first, it leads to vaccine hesitancy, defined here as the delay in acceptance or the refusal of vaccination despite the availability of vaccines through national programs (MacDonald, 2015, p. 4163) and, second, when this vaccine hesitancy ultimately undermines the effectiveness of vaccination programs and threatens the health of individuals and populations. At the same time, these controversies surrounding vaccination reflect the diversity of moral and epistemic views that characterize plural societies. Hence, the normative question this book seeks to answer is as follows:

> How should a constitutional liberal-democratic government deal with deep controversies concerning vaccination, given the fact that these may lead to vaccine hesitancy, which can subsequently pose a genuine threat to public health? If encouragement of voluntary participation in vaccination programs is not sufficient, can coercive measures be justified—and, if so, under what conditions?

We take for granted the broad consensus in the biomedical and epidemiological sciences that vaccines as used in collective programs are effective in preventing disease and that they can be safely used; moreover, on a population level, these vaccines have a very positive risk–benefit ratio (Dudley et al., 2020). We also endorse the general idea that government policy on infectious diseases should be based on state-of-the-art biomedical and epidemiological evidence. At the same time, discussions and the antivaccination movement emerging at the time of writing make it clear that there are evident epistemic and moral disputes about these issues that cannot simply be pushed aside by appealing to a scientific and professional consensus. Indeed, the very aim of this book is to discuss the regulation of childhood vaccination in the face of these disputes.

Two caveats apply. The focus on affluent liberal-democratic societies does not imply that we think that vaccination policies—and the ethical questions they raise—in less affluent countries are less important. On the contrary: low- and middle-income countries face much higher mortality rates due to infectious diseases. Nevertheless, this book explicitly engages with the current discussion of vaccine hesitancy in pluralistic democracies. The problem of vaccine hesitancy might also be relevant in other countries, including many low- and middle-income ones, but we think that in those contexts, the question of how to deal with pluralism is vastly overshadowed by the absence or scarcity of basic public health infrastructures and by the inequitable access to health care and vaccinations.[6] This generates important discussions, for example, on vaccine nationalism and the unilateral actions of affluent countries to provide their own populations with access to vaccines ahead of other countries, which deprives low- and middle-income countries of access to vaccines—as has become very clear during the COVID-19 pandemic (Gruszczynski & Wu, 2021; Katz et al., 2021). We acknowledge the importance of these global justice debates, but in the context of this book, we seek to engage with a different discussion.

The second caveat is that our focus on vaccine hesitancy may suggest that it is a widespread phenomenon in liberal democracies. This is not the case. Vaccinating is still the norm; large majorities in most countries participate voluntarily and wholeheartedly. The discussion is about the ragged edges: the small part that categorically opposes vaccination and the somewhat larger group of parents that is on the fence. The problem is that for some diseases, the vaccination rate must be very high to prevent outbreaks, and even a relatively small percentage of vaccine refusers can undermine societal protection against vaccine-preventable diseases.

In the next two chapters, we set the stage for our analysis by discussing state responsibilities and policy options, and by exploring objections against vaccination and the grounds for respecting those objections in a liberal democracy. Subsequently, we develop a principled argument for liberty-limiting vaccination policies that is largely based on John Stuart Mill's *On Liberty* (chapters 4 and 5), and we explore contextual factors that are decisive in the justification of specific immunization policies, targeting children (chapters 6 and 7) and adults (chapter 8). In the last part of the book, we discuss how public health authorities can be trustworthy in times when many dispute the scientific evidence on which immunization policies are built, and we offer a critical reflection on our appeals to John Stuart Mill's liberal philosophy.

2 The Role of Government in Promoting Collective Immunization

The central question in this book is how governments should regulate vaccination, given their role in protecting individual and population health, that herd immunity is an important collective good, and that not all citizens endorse vaccination for themselves or their children. A first step in our normative analysis, then, is to ask whether national governments have a role at all in promoting vaccinations. In this chapter, we distinguish various grounds on which liberal-democratic states can organize collective immunization. In the last part of this chapter, we outline the various modalities the government can use to promote collective immunization.

2.1 The Responsibility of Government: Protecting Public Health and Societal Life

As the COVID-19 pandemic has made abundantly clear, an infectious disease can spread rapidly in a population, causing illness and premature death. Disease outbreaks can be a major, and potentially disruptive, threat to society. They involve not only the morbidity and mortality themselves but also the threat of a disease and the fear it can generate of being infected by others, in private or public, that can affect—or, in extreme cases, paralyze—social coexistence. Contagious diseases may, therefore, directly undermine social interaction and community. The large-scale lockdowns following the 2020 COVID-19 outbreak were implemented because there was not yet a vaccine or another way to protect society and its members against the disease. But well-known vaccine-preventable diseases like measles can also reemerge and disrupt social life on a smaller scale, for example, in schools or childcare centers, and can put health care systems under serious pressure.

For these reasons, combatting infectious diseases is generally considered a classic task for government, especially if those diseases transmit from person to person and infections occur in societal life. The paradox of infectious disease control is that in response to (an immediate threat of) an outbreak, the protection of a community often requires measures that impose restrictions on social contact, including social distancing, isolation, or quarantine. In the past few decades, most people in affluent countries have only learned of such large outbreaks via historical documents or portrayals in novels. Philip Roth's novel *Nemesis* (2010), for example, provides a dramatic story of the impact of a 1944 emerging polio epidemic in Newark (New Jersey) on children and parents. Even though current vaccination levels will often preclude the devastating impact that epidemics had before the introduction of vaccines, outbreaks of childhood diseases still can and do disrupt societal life, not only through the impact of a disease and the collective fear of infection but also through the public health responses implemented to contain or mitigate the spread of a disease.

For younger generations, the COVID-19 pandemic has been an acute firsthand experience of the impact of a large disease outbreak. After the first cases in China, which were contained by a complete lockdown, a major outbreak occurred in northern Italy in February 2020. Hospitals were overwhelmed with patients with lung disease, and intensive care departments appeared unable to offer mechanical ventilation to everyone who needed it. Within weeks, the disease was everywhere in the world, especially hitting nursing home residents and older people more generally, but younger people—including many health care workers—also fell ill. When it became clear that initial quarantine and isolation measures were insufficient, complete regions and ultimately countries went into lockdown. Borders were closed, flights were cancelled, and schools and universities closed, and in many places, citizens were only allowed to leave their homes for necessary reasons. Not all countries faced a situation as bad as northern Italy did, but often hospitals were overwhelmed or could only just deal with the large influx of patients. Health care for non-COVID-19 issues was reduced to a minimum to prioritize the victims of the pandemic. Large parts of the global economy came to a standstill, and the expectation was that economic losses would lead to much more suffering in the years to come.

By mid-2020, China and, later, Europe had slowly recovered from the first wave of the pandemic, but infections in other parts of the world, notably

North and South America, were surging. As a result, new waves of the pandemic emerged, and lockdowns had to be reinstated. The world awaited impatiently the advent of novel vaccines to fight the disease. But even after the arrival of the vaccines and the massive rollout of vaccination programs, it remained hard to keep COVID-19 infections in check, because the vaccine did not fully protect against the spread of the disease, and vaccination rates remained suboptimal.

Such an epidemic outbreak first and foremost affects society by overwhelming the capacity of hospital care—in particular, the availability of intensive care units (ICUs). This implies that fewer staff will be available for other patients, complete hospital wards may need to be reserved for infected patients, and special (time- and energy-consuming) precautions need to be taken to prevent those infections from spreading to other patients in the hospital. Of course, the capacity of hospitals and ICUs is geared to a steady flow of patients, but a characteristic of outbreaks of infectious diseases is that they generate waves of patients, most likely during the winter months. Moreover, patients with COVID-19 remain in ICU wards for a relatively long time, usually two weeks or more, which generates a major drain on ICU capacity. At the same time, sufficient ICU capacity is not a frivolous luxury. Anyone, at any time, can get involved in a serious traffic accident, have a heart attack, or encounter another acute health problem.

Obviously, not every outbreak of an infectious disease disrupts society so thoroughly. Yet it is clear that epidemics of vaccine-preventable diseases, notably COVID-19, but also polio and measles, can threaten and undermine societal life in a myriad of ways. This is a central concern for any government, liberal, socialist, or conservative, and the concern is consistent with diverging political philosophies. Even libertarians who plead for a minimal role of the state might accept that governments have a basic task to protect society against external and internal threats.[1] A major part of the legal framework governing infectious disease control can be justified in this way. Protection against outbreaks is a basic condition for a flourishing and open society, and in many cases, vaccination and robust herd immunity will offer such protection most effectively, because they prevent outbreaks altogether. Moreover, collective immunization makes it possible for people to trust that, in normal circumstances, being part of a crowd, sneezing, laughing, and even talking do not create severe health risks. If liberalism and other views that leave only a relatively modest role for the state can accept that the state still has a responsibility to protect the basic functioning of society by creating conditions in which people can live together safely without constant fear of dangerous infections, this will arguably also be the case for egalitarian or utilitarian political philosophies that favor a more expansive role for governments in promoting health. This justifies the conclusion that most if not all political views support the belief that a liberal-democratic state has a responsibility to do all that is reasonable to prevent outbreaks of contagious diseases.

2.2   The Benefits of National Immunization Programs

Immunization is a highly effective intervention that can prevent contagious diseases while still allowing people to engage in social life. Vaccination programs can effectively reduce infection risks and, more specifically, prevent or at least limit the impact of outbreaks. The latter effect, however, requires a large part of the population to be immunized. Just offering individuals the possibility of getting vaccinated might not be enough; from the perspective of the governmental responsibility to prevent outbreaks, it is important to aim at group-level protection.

To realize this, vaccination against such infectious diseases should not merely be discussed in terms of the individual health of the vaccinated person. It should also be analyzed in terms of *public health*, and that explains the additional importance of coordinated national immunization programs. By offering vaccinations collectively and striving toward a high coverage that is sufficient for herd protection, it becomes almost impossible for disease-causing microorganisms to reproduce and circulate within a population, and small outbreaks will soon fade out. The benefits of vaccination programs thus surpass the aggregate benefits for all individual vaccinated persons. Herd immunity protects several categories of vulnerable persons who cannot be protected individually against a disease. The first category consists of infants and young children who have not yet completed the recommended immunization schedule. A clear example is the potential risk of exposure to measles for children aged between six and fourteen months. In their first months after birth, infants still benefit from the immunity they have acquired from their mother. After six months, this protection fades away, but these children will not receive their first MMR vaccination before the age of twelve to fourteen months.[2] If there is robust herd immunity, this temporary lack of individual immunity is unproblematic: the chance that these children will be exposed to the virus is negligible. The second category of vulnerability concerns persons whose vaccination turns out to be insufficiently effective because it does not mount an adequate immune response. In the case of measles, the first of two vaccinations, administered around the fourteenth month, provides an average protection of 95 percent. Adding a second inoculation around the age of nine years results in an average protection of 96 percent (Di Pietrantonj et al., 2020). This means that 4 to 5 percent of vaccinated persons remain vulnerable to the disease. And even persons for whom the vaccine has initially worked well can become vulnerable if their immune system is weakened due to illness or immune-suppressive medical treatment. The third category concerns those who cannot undergo vaccination for medical reasons: because they have a particular form (or forms) of cancer, have a compromised immune system, or are likely to have a serious allergic reaction. The final category of vulnerable persons consists of children whose parents have refrained from vaccinating them. In all these cases, exposure to a pathogen would create a risk that is prevented by robust herd immunity. It is through this collective protection that large-scale vaccination programs are so much more effective than individual vaccination. This is the reason why collective vaccination programs are cornerstones of public health programs in liberal democracies.

In addition, maintaining herd immunity within a country not only benefits the population of that country itself. It also inhibits the spread of infection worldwide and could thus contribute to the eradication of a disease altogether. This is a significant feature, even if, arguably, most programs primarily aim at controlling the disease domestically to protect the health of that nation. However, infectious diseases do not respect national borders. Moreover, mortality and morbidity caused by infectious diseases are almost always higher in low- and middle-income countries due to poverty, inadequate nutrition, and relatively weak health care infrastructures. If global immunization rates remain high, all countries are contributing to the protection of people who live in conditions that make infections most dangerous (WHO, 2013).

To conclude, collective immunization that succeeds in establishing and maintaining group-level protection can be considered serving a public good that is beneficial to all persons: young or old, ill or healthy, vaccinated or not, or whether they like it or not. All of them benefit from the prevention of outbreaks that may cause severe disease and potentially disrupt societal life. Given that protection from infectious diseases is a core responsibility of society, governments have an important task in organizing national immunization programs that aim at high vaccination rates.

2.3   The Responsibility of Government: Ensuring Equitable Access to Vaccinations

As important as the collective benefits of vaccination may be, the protective effects can only be attained via the individuals who are immunized. Immunization first and foremost renders individual benefits. Some vaccines do not even result in group protection, as they protect against diseases that do not spread from human to human—tetanus, for example. Other vaccines, such as the HPV vaccination, do result in group protection, but their function is not to protect against sudden outbreaks of a disease: the cancers caused by HPV infections do not manifest themselves in acute outbreaks but in individual, unconnected instances. Some might argue that the government has no responsibility to make those individual benefits available.[3] Yet even if we disregard for the moment the public good of herd protection, we can still see immunization as a key element of public health care. In public health ethics—and notably in the ethical literature on universal health insurance—justice is seen as argument *par excellence* that supports the state taking responsibility for health care. Health has a special value for each individual as it is a central feature of human well-being that also influences what people can become and do in their lives and the extent to which they can employ the benefits of their fundamental rights (Wilson, 2021). Disease and disability, on the other hand, can strongly constrain their mobility, their ability to earn an income, and their potential to live according to their idea of the good life. Health care therefore has an important—sometimes essential—function to protect people's range of opportunities. In a liberal-democratic state, citizens are due equal concern, and this supports policies that ensure that everyone has access to (at least basic) health care provisions. In his Rawlsian approach to health justice, Norman Daniels sees equal access to basic health care as a matter of fair equality of opportunity (Daniels, 2001). In a capabilitarian approach, one can expect health to fulfill a central role, either as one of the basic human capabilities (Nussbaum, 1992) or as a meta-capability that is necessary to have access to all other central capabilities (Venkatapuram,

2011). And again, for most people, access to health care is a necessary condition for protecting these capabilities. Although the idea of equal access to essential health care may not fit well in libertarian political philosophies, it is widely accepted, and indeed, almost all high-income countries—maybe with the US as the most notable exception—have some form of universal health care coverage (Garrett et al., 2009).

This is not the place to provide a profound justification of the role of democratic states in realizing equitable access to health care, but *if* we assume that there is such a role for government, then there is no reason to limit this idea to patient care and to not also include certain forms of preventive care, especially vaccination. To promote fair equality of opportunity, the state should create equal access to vaccinations that are necessary for individual persons to maintain health. If particular persons run a substantial risk of developing a severe disease and vaccination can take away or significantly reduce the risk, it is unfair if some of them can afford vaccination and others cannot. If this is the case, the state has moral reasons to offer equal access to this vaccination—within the limits of reasonable health care expenditures, of course.

Let us take vaccination against human papillomavirus (HPV) as an example. HPV is a sexually transmittable infection that mostly occurs without clinical symptoms and often disappears over time. However, if the infection perseveres, it may cause various forms of cancer in genital and oral body parts. HPV is responsible for most cases of cervical cancer, one of the most common forms of cancer in high- as well as low- and middle-income countries. The possibility of sexually transmitted HPV infections is arguably not an immediate threat to public health or societal life, because the ensuing cancers do not manifest themselves in acute, massive outbreaks. Governments therefore have no compelling reason to offer vaccination as part of their responsibility to protect societal life. Moreover, in high-income countries that have universal health care coverage, presumably all women who are diagnosed with cervical cancer will be eligible for treatment. Yet, given that both the disease and the treatment come with heavy burdens and risks, and that the success of treatment is limited, a vaccination that reduces a woman's risk of developing cervical cancer by 80 percent or more makes a huge difference (Laprise et al., 2020). If such protection were only available to women who can afford to pay for the vaccinations, this may well be a matter of inequity. Hence, even if there was no clear justification (utilitarian or otherwise) for offering vaccination in terms of protecting society, it may still be ethically appropriate for reasons of justice. Governments can also decide to aim at herd immunity against HPV. This would involve vaccinating girls *and* boys. Males will also benefit from HPV vaccination—it offers protection against genital and anal cancers. The risk of developing these diseases is very slim, though, which implies that the individual health benefits of HPV vaccination for boys are only remote. HPV vaccination of boys can thus be justified by an appeal to the public good of herd immunity—primarily to protect women against cervical cancer—but it will be more difficult to argue that boys should be offered vaccination as a matter of equitable access to essential preventive health care.

Whether a specific vaccination *is* considered an element of basic health care that should be available to everyone and what criteria should guide such ethical choices will be a matter of political deliberation. This concerns, for example, discussions about which vaccines are included in collective programs and which are left out. The harmful impact of some vaccine-preventable diseases, such as measles and polio, is so far beyond dispute that vaccinations against them are included in all programs. The argument is less obvious for other vaccines. For example, some but not all countries have included the varicella vaccination for children: in the Netherlands, it was decided that the disease burden of varicella was not large enough (Gezondheidsraad, 2020; Pierik, 2020a). It might be difficult to attain consensus on what preventive interventions are to be made available for everyone given the need to contain rising health care costs and given that many people might be tempted to prioritize therapy for patients in acute need above vaccinations that have less tangible effects on individual persons (Verweij, 2015). On the other hand, policies aiming at justice in relation to health cannot do without adequate preventive care, and vaccination programs are certainly among the most effective preventive strategies.

Another line of justice-based reasoning addresses the government's special responsibilities toward children and their vaccination. The state's responsibility for promoting and protecting the health of adult individuals is limited. It should at least not undermine each person's own responsibility for their health and allow individuals to make their own health-related choices. Yet this assumption about there being specific limits to government responsibility for health can apply only to competent adults who are to be respected as autonomous persons—it does not apply to children who cannot yet make responsible autonomous choices. Moreover, emphasizing the responsibility of individual adults can only be fair if they have achieved a basic level of health in their childhood years and a capability to maintain it afterward. Universal childhood vaccination programs can play an important role in that respect. This suggests that governments have a special responsibility to ensure the health of children, first because children cannot take that responsibility themselves and second because such programs offer children—at least in some respects—an equal basis on which to achieve and maintain health for the rest of their lives.

Note that these considerations of justice do not primarily focus on achieving or maintaining a public good such as the protection of *public* health and the conditions for societal life—they are ultimately about ensuring and promoting the health of every individual. Hence, considerations made in this and previous sections jointly acknowledge that vaccination policies yield collective as well as individual benefits and that the state has responsibilities regarding both.

2.4   National Immunization Programs: Mapping the Legal Regimes

A large variety of possible legal regimes may govern vaccination programs for children and adults. In this section, we distinguish several categories and describe options in more detail. One option, only presented for the sake of comprehensiveness, is that a government has no policy whatsoever regarding vaccination. The decision to vaccinate would then be left completely to individuals, either in their role of an individual recipient or as a parent, and a government would not encourage or discourage any choice. It might even be the case that citizens have to pay for their vaccinations themselves. However, given the fact that protection against infectious diseases is generally considered such an important, even classic, government task, all states, in one way or another, promote or even mandate childhood immunization against at least some diseases.

In box 2.1, we present a general overview of policies that are available to stimulate both childhood vaccination and vaccination for adults.[4] Since vaccination programs during the past few decades have primarily targeted children, most of the examples presented below revolve around childhood

Box 2.1

Degrees of Coercion in Vaccination Policies

Voluntary policies: encouraging

information campaigns

offer vaccinations free of charge, easy to access, adequate reminders

persuasive communication; positive nudges

offer opportunities for persons not vaccinated in their youth to catch up later

allow childcare centers or schools to publish vaccination rates

Voluntary policies: norm expressing

require childcare centers or schools to publish vaccination rates

opt-out policy: parents must take action if they choose to avoid vaccination

allow childcare centers and schools to refuse unvaccinated children

expand possibilities for tort cases in case someone is infected by an unvaccinated person

Mandatory policies

set vaccination as a condition for child benefits

require that all children attending child day care centers are vaccinated (with/without exemptions)

require that all children attending schools are vaccinated (with exemptions)

Compulsory policies

require that all children in schools are vaccinated, without exemptions, and back this up with financial penalties

make vaccine refusal a criminal offense with punitive sanctions

Enforced vaccination

impose vaccination with force (i.e., against the will of a person or their parent) vaccination. We distinguish categories of policies (encouraging, norm expressing, mandatory, compulsory by law, enforced by law) that involve different degrees of coercion.

2.4.1 Voluntary Policies

Encouraging people to be vaccinated or to have their children immunized can be done in multiple ways that can also be combined to render them more effective. Initially, a government can launch campaigns to inform the public about the dangers of infectious diseases and the benefits and limited risks of vaccination, as an antidote to antivaccination websites.[5] Most governments also promote access to immunization by making it available free of charge and by securing sufficient supply. An obvious way to encourage participation is to make it as easy as possible, for example, sending invitations and reminders when necessary and making vaccination sites easily accessible. In addition, another way of encouraging hesitant persons is to visit them in their neighborhood or at home with information and the opportunity to receive the vaccination on the spot. The Dutch government, for example, entices parents to vaccinate their children through active invitations and an effective system of vaccination reminders. Parents can ignore the schedule if they want to, but the program generates an unmistakable message that will make it highly unlikely that appointments are overlooked.

In addition, the government can allow and enable day care centers and schools to publicize their nonvaccination rates. This provides parents with relevant information to be taken into consideration, along with other variables, when they are choosing a specific day care center or school: travel distance, pedagogic climate, opening hours, price, and so on.[6]

Note, however, that even in high-income countries (e.g., in rural parts of the US or in some countries in Europe), access to vaccines is not self-evident. Unfortunately, public health institutions are not always well funded, so getting one's child vaccinated may be burdensome for parents (e.g., require traveling a long distance) even if vaccines are free of charge. It goes without saying that access to vaccination should be optimal before more coercive policies are adopted.

2.4.2 Norm-Expressing Voluntary Policies

Normative policies go a step further in the sense that they do not just facilitate and encourage choosing immunization but also make it the norm or express it as such—without immediately enforcing parents to comply. They could *require* childcare centers to publish vaccination rates rather than just allowing them to do so. Childcare centres could even be given the option to deny unvaccinated children access. It is clear that this strongly *expresses* the norm that children should be vaccinated, without it actually being legally enforced. It may create clarity for people who are seeking a safe environment for their children, but it does not come without risk. Arguably, some schools or childcare centers that do not require vaccination may end up with a population in which almost no children have been immunized, which would be a perfect context for outbreaks of infectious diseases (Pierik & Verweij, 2019b). These types of regulations will probably not only influence parental decision-making in the sense that they create choices but also have an impact on public opinion and may even lead to polarization about childhood vaccinations in a way that means parents will experience social pressure to opt for vaccination.

Another normative approach would be to organize the program in such a way that *opting in* is the default position, and parents must take action if they want to *opt out* (Opel & Omer, 2015). For example, opting out is only possible if parents first visit their family physician to discuss the reasons for their choice—so the physician can question incorrect assumptions or resolve unnecessary concerns. In New Zealand, parents must show an immunization certificate signed by their doctor at the early childcare service or school. The physician will sign the certificate if parents have made a well-considered choice to opt out, and in this way, the policy prevents parents forgetting to have their child vaccinated or forgoing vaccination because of the burden of visiting their physician (Ministry of Health, 2020, pp. 611–612). The policy ensures that seeking vaccination is not more burdensome for parents than waiving the shots.[7]

2.4.3 Mandatory Policies

Policies that take a step further are what we call mandatory policies, the name implying even more clearly that the government expects all children to be immunized. We define *mandatory vaccination* programs as those programs in which the state withholds valuable social goods or services from persons who choose to forgo vaccination for themselves or their child for nonmedical reasons.

A very specific example of mandatory vaccination was imposed during the COVID-19 pandemic: people had to show proof of vaccination to get access to restaurants or other social or cultural activities. Mandatory policies have been much more common in relation to childhood immunization. For example, in Australia, immunization is a requirement for child-related advantages, including child allowance: the *no jab no play* policy and the *no jab no pay* policy. The former is a federal program focusing on a national entitlement scheme, while the latter is a set of distinct state-level policies (Attwell et al., 2020a; Beard et al., 2017; Leask & Danchin, 2017). Parents who do not fully immunize their children—up to nineteen years of age—will cease to be eligible for various forms of family assistance payments. This policy leaves the decision regarding vaccination to parents, but if they decide to forgo vaccination, this will lead to various financial setbacks.[8]

Another mandatory policy is requiring all children in childcare centers to participate in the national immunization program and therefore receiving all the age-appropriate immunizations. Parents can still opt out by organizing other forms of care for their child. In many countries, including the United States, Italy, and France, children must have completed their vaccination schedule before they are allowed in schools. There may be various ways for parents to opt out, either by homeschooling their children or by applying for an exemption. Many US states also offer parents the possibility of being exempted from vaccinating their child for religious and/or philosophical reasons. We will discuss exemptions in more detail in chapter 6. Interestingly, the various US states differ regarding the extent to which they allow or discourage such nonmedical exemptions (Navin & Largent, 2017). So even if a completed childhood vaccination scheme is a requirement for day care or school entry, there are still degrees of power a state can use and apply to enforce the policy.

2.4.4 Compulsory Policies

A further coercive step is to impose a legal duty on parents or other citizens to vaccinate. We define *compulsory vaccination* as policies that make vaccine refusal a criminal or administrative offense, backed up with punishment such as a fine or imprisonment. The punishment can be directly linked to vaccine refusal (e.g., in Belgium, refusal to have one's child vaccinated against polio can be punished with imprisonment) or indirectly by punishing parents because they refuse to fulfill the requirements for compulsory school attendance of their child.[9]

2.4.5 Forced Immunization Policies

The most far-reaching intervention would be *forced immunization*, which involves vaccination against the parents' will. This could be done through the temporary suspension of the exercise of parental authority, during which the child can be vaccinated. This bypasses parents' choice completely by eliminating their opportunity to avoid or forgo the measure. Such a measure would be extreme, but it might make sense if unprotected children run an immediate risk (e.g., during an outbreak), as we will discuss in section 5.4.

2.5 The Intervention Ladder

Our taxonomy of legal regimes can be considered an application of the *intervention ladder* that the Nuffield Council on Bioethics (2007) proposed for the ethical review of public health measures. The intervention ladder is based on the assumption that compulsory or mandatory policies can only be justified if less intrusive measures have been exhausted or are expected to have an insufficient effect. Compulsory policies, then, would only be considered a last resort. At the same time, governments are obliged to ensure effective protection and to take precautions against (outbreaks of) infectious diseases, and this may well offer a sufficient basis for mandatory policies. Determining which "rung" of the intervention ladder is appropriate for a particular society at a specific moment ultimately depends on contextual factors like the level of vaccine coverage, the risk of outbreaks, and the severity of specific diseases. At the same time, it may often not be easy to rank all possible measures along one ladder. For example, in the United States, all states have mandatory vaccination policies, but how easy it is for parents to be exempted can differ. In fact, a mandatory policy requiring vaccination for school entry from which it is easy to gain an exemption may be not more "intrusive" in practice than a fully voluntary "opt-out" policy. As we will argue in the later chapters, governments need a strong justification for immunization policies that go beyond voluntary choice. They should invest a great deal of energy in encouraging the acceptance of policies and should only revert to the enforcement of legal duties as a last resort when voluntary policies cease to protect the basic interests of the children involved. This is because liberty is such a central value in a constitutional liberal democracy.[10]

Indeed, it is vital for achieving the public good of herd immunity that a large majority wholeheartedly accepts vaccination and is willing to cooperate in collective immunization schemes. The success of policies that offer collective protection against diseases is determined not only by the quality of vaccines provided but also by the amount of trust that the public has in the health care system and health care professionals, where trust implies "deferring with comfort and confidence to others, about something beyond our knowledge or power, in ways that can potentially hurt us" (Whyte and Crease, as quoted in Goldenberg, 2016, p. 570). The importance of public trust sets limits on the level of coercion that the state can use to promote immunization. We will return to trust and trustworthiness in chapter 9.

2.6 The Role of Government in Promoting Collective Immunization: A Conclusion

In this chapter, we established that the state has a responsibility to protect the conditions that are necessary for a well-functioning society, and also a duty to guarantee equitable access to essential vaccinations for every citizen. These tasks normally coincide. National immunization programs aim at high vaccination rates, and this will likely also promote equitable access. Such protection is a fundamental interest of each and every citizen and a precondition for the enjoyment of fundamental rights for both children and adults. In the forthcoming chapters, we discuss in what ways this may involve policies that constrain the freedom of individuals to refuse vaccination. This will often be about vaccine-preventable childhood diseases, but if there is a threat of society-disrupting outbreaks or even pandemics, like COVID-19, there is a particular need to consider whether coercive vaccination of adult citizens can be justified as well.

Most infectious diseases affect populations primarily via children, because their immune system has not yet encountered the pathogens causing the various diseases. Moreover, since children are too young to make an independent and well-considered choice about vaccination, others—their parents or the government—should make this decision for them, guided by the best interests of the child. In a modern democracy, it seems rather obvious that it is the parents who will authorize medical treatment of their child—including vaccination. But what if parents decline (some of) the vaccinations that the state considers to be necessary to protect public health? In chapters 4 through 7, we develop an argument about how liberal-democratic governments should deal with such disputes. We argue in favor of contextual childhood vaccination policies that upscale interference: programs are voluntary when possible, but they are changed to a mandatory (or even compulsory) approach when that is necessary to maintain the herd immunity required to protect children's basic interests.

The responsibility of the government to protect public health is not limited to childhood immunization. Outbreaks of novel life-threatening contagious diseases can endanger a well-functioning society in a myriad of ways. They affect health and threaten the lives of many, can lead to an overwhelmed health care system, and can result in a fear of infection that will inhibit societal—economic and educational—life. Moreover, the necessary public health responses for reducing social proximity, gathering, interaction, and so on will add further to the societal disruption. In chapter 8, we argue that in such a context, if a safe and effective vaccine is available, governments are justified in curtailing the freedom of citizens who refuse vaccinations—and this will often not only be about immunization of children but especially also of adults.

In all cases, however, vaccination refusal and the grounds that individuals invoke to forgo immunization should be taken seriously. Let us explore this in the next chapter.

3   Forgoing Vaccination: Reasons and Rights

Since the introduction of the first large-scale programs at the beginning of the nineteenth century, vaccination has become both a lauded and a controversial phenomenon. Most parents voluntarily enroll their children in such programs because they are convinced of the beneficial effect of vaccination on the health of their children. But a significant percentage of citizens remain unwilling to accept vaccination for themselves or their children—even when there is a clear threat such as COVID-19. This chapter discusses the various causes of vaccine hesitancy: the delay in acceptance or refusal of vaccinations that are available and easily accessible through national programs. Some objections to immunization are embedded in a comprehensive secular or religious view of life, while others fit in a more rationalistic perspective. In the upcoming sections, we present and discuss three types of reasons that some groups of people have for objecting to vaccination. These reasons may crosscut each other, so our taxonomy of reasons can be considered a heuristic separation of partly overlapping perspectives.[1]

In the second part of this chapter (from section 3.5 onward), we argue that in a pluralistic democratic state, these objections should not simply be ignored by the government; instead it should, to a large extent, respect citizens' freedom to make their own choices about accepting or rejecting preventive options for themselves and, to some extent, for their children.

3.1   Religious Opposition to Vaccination: Divine Providence

The first category of vaccine objections is of a clearly religious nature: it concerns persons who are convinced that vaccination interferes with divine providence or that a disease is a spiritual phenomenon that should be healed or prevented through prayer instead of medication. Examples are concerns endorsed in specific Protestant Christian congregations, notably in the Netherlands and the US. One of the most perseverant types of groups that oppose vaccination are "pietistic reformed groups" (*bevindelijk gereformeerden*): orthodox Protestant communities in the Netherlands, consisting of about 250,000 members (Ruijs, 2012, pp. 7–24; van der Meiden, 1993, pp. 60–72; Zwemer, 2001, pp. 14–19). They believe that God has predestined the fate and therefore also health and illness of all human beings. They are aware of the risks of vaccine-preventable disease and disease outbreaks, will fear the possible negative health effects for themselves or their children, and might fully acknowledge the medical effectiveness of immunization. Nevertheless, they oppose vaccination for themselves and their children because they prioritize their religious values and faith in God over the medical benefits of immunization. Taking divine providence as a starting point, vaccination could be considered an "inappropriate meddling in the work of God." Moreover, immunization would be evidence of a lack of trust in God and a refusal to submit to divine discipline or punishment. Such arguments are usually supported by references to Matthew 9:12: "It is not the healthy who need a doctor, but the sick." This quote suggests a categorical distinction between medical prevention and therapy. The former is prohibited while the latter is allowed. A somewhat different attitude is common among Christian Scientists in North America. They argue that disease is a spiritual rather than a material phenomenon that should be healed through prayer rather than by medical interventions. Members of this religious community refuse vaccines because they believe that physical illness is an illusion of the material world and that prayer can help us to correct the false beliefs that give rise to illness (Colgrove, 2005). A further religious objection that is sometimes invoked is that research on or production of certain vaccines would have involved the use of cell lines derived from aborted fetuses (Giubilini et al., 2021).

From an epidemiological perspective, it is relevant that these religious groups often live in tightly knit and geographically concentrated communities that are sometimes even relatively closed. As a result, vaccine coverage in these communities and villages will be very low, creating conditions for infectious diseases to spread rapidly within the group (Ruijs, 2012, pp. 136–148). Indeed, in the past few decades, the so-called Bible Belt region in the Netherlands has seen various outbreaks of polio (1971, 1978, 1992), measles (2000, 2013), and rubella (2004). It is clear that members of these religious congregations usually have very strong and principled objections against vaccination.[2] And even though they may deplore the possible health risks for their children, they postulate that their fate—whether or not they are infected with measles—is ultimately in God's hands and that humans should not meddle with divine providence through vaccination.

3.2 Anthroposophist Objections: Diseases Contribute to Development

The second group of objections centers on the assumption that certain childhood diseases have a beneficial role in the physical, mental, and spiritual development of children. This idea is based on the philosophy of anthroposophy as formulated by Rudolf Steiner (1861–1925), which is especially endorsed in some regions in South Germany and Switzerland. As an educational philosophy, anthroposophy is prominent in over a thousand Waldorf schools all over the world (Navin, 2016, pp. 117–120). Many people in these communities also embrace anthroposophical approaches to medicine (Bartelme, 2020). There is no formalized policy on immunization within the practice of anthroposophist medicine. However, the basic assumption is that a disease such as measles is seen as a relatively innocent but necessary struggle in the process of a child's development into an adult—on par with losing primary teeth. The anthroposophist doctrine explains that such childhood diseases provide individuals with a natural resilience against diseases like cancer and allergies later in life. Measles and some other childhood diseases are seen as innocent and beneficial, so followers of Steiner's anthroposophy prefer their children to encounter rather than avoid these infections. Medical practitioners should therefore not prevent this through vaccination but instead should help the patient to deal with the illness. Arthur Allen quotes a parent of a child in a Waldorf school:

> There's a little bit of soulfulness with getting ill. . . . Sometimes people say that after a fever you see a difference in a child's being. It really strengthens them. . . . [People who vaccinate their children] never allow them the soulfulness of being ill. (Allen, 2007, p. 351)

This is why some families seek to expose their young children to infections rather than prevent such exposure by means of vaccination. They even organize so-called measles parties—*to put spots on tots*. Although followers of Steiner's anthroposophy might not live in communities that are as close as those of the Protestant religious groups discussed in the previous section, their often unvaccinated children probably do go to the same Waldorf schools, childcare centers, and summer camps. This can result in local unvaccinated pockets, as noted previously, in an otherwise robust herd immunity, and outbreaks of measles and other vaccine-preventable diseases in anthroposophist schools or school camps are not uncommon.

3.3   Concerns about Risks and Benefits: Autism and Beyond

The third category of objections to vaccination is raised by people who suspect that the risks of vaccination outweigh the purported benefits. It is not strange for parents to be concerned about potential adverse effects of a vaccine for their child, but for the past two decades or so these worries are also actively promoted and spread by a vocal movement in which many members can be seen as being *antivaccination*. They convey their message through social media, books, websites, and documentaries. It is a multifaceted movement that includes "spiritual" or "holistic" approaches, adherents of "natural healing" and "alternative healing," and those who oppose employing "nonnatural" means of promoting one's health. Their critique of vaccination is sometimes embedded in a more encompassing view of life, like anthroposophy, a "back to nature philosophy," or the idea that one's body is a temple or otherwise sacred. But it might also find support in more down-to-earth sociopolitical sentiments like a lack of trust in government, public health authorities, scientific institutions, and "Big Pharma." The different perspectives find one another in their shared critique of the ways governments organize and promote large-scale vaccination programs. Unlike religious groups, which are primarily inwardly oriented, antivaccination movements actively and successfully reach out to young parents, sometimes with the help of celebrities and often by stimulating parents to "do their own research" rather than following the advice of mainstream medicine.

An important event that has worked as a catalyst for this modern antivaccination movement is the *MMR-vaccine-causes-autism* controversy that was triggered by the publication of an article by Andrew Wakefield and coauthors in *The Lancet* (1998). Wakefield presented a study that suggested a link between the MMR (measles, mumps, rubella) triple vaccine, bowel disease, and autism. The link was widely reported in the media and led to societal unrest and a sharp decline in MMR vaccine uptake in the UK and other countries. As a result, measles outbreaks started to rise again. The controversy generated a huge industry of peer-reviewed studies, none of which could corroborate the alleged vaccination–autism link (Jain et al., 2015; Taylor et al., 2014). *The Lancet* retracted the article in 2010 because it was discovered that the study was based on fraudulent data and because Wakefield appeared to have had undisclosed financial interests in establishing a link with autism and bowel disease (Deer, 2011a, 2011b). Soon afterward, Wakefield was struck off the medical register and thus banned from practicing medicine in the UK. Wakefield's claim has been fully debunked in medical science, but the suggested link between the vaccine and autism remains "the most damaging medical hoax of the last 100 years" (Flaherty, 2011, p. 1302). Antivaccination groups and even some politicians continue to accept and repeat it as if it is a matter of fact.

Many vaccine critics seek to carve out "all-natural" lives for themselves and their children, to maintain "purity" or avoid contamination. They point to allegedly toxic substances, either the vaccine itself or adjuvants that play a role in creating a stronger immune response or that are used to preserve the vaccine. Others argue that current programs overwhelm a child's immune system because it is forced to handle too many vaccines too early in life (Biss, 2014).

All in all, even if there is ample biomedical and epidemiological evidence about the safety of vaccines in such collective programs, parents may well have doubts and remain hesitant about vaccination. Like all medicines, vaccines can also have side effects. Even when all reasonable precautions are taken in the manufacture and delivery of vaccinations, it is inevitable that adverse reactions occur. Most side effects are local, minor, and unavoidable. The purpose of vaccination is to elicit a response from the immune system, and this is often accompanied by temporary symptoms. These symptoms indicate that the vaccine is doing its work, emulating infection, inducing the requisite immune response by the body, and building protection against the disease for which the vaccine is a proxy. Major harmful effects that can be causally linked to the vaccine are exceptionally rare nowadays. For example, the live oral polio vaccine can cause paralytic polio in very rare cases, and this has been a reason for most countries to switch to the inactivated injectable vaccine. Such major adverse effects are extremely rare for the vaccines used in current collective programs.

It is not hard to understand that parents worry about vaccines and the risk of side effects, given that most vaccine-preventable diseases have become virtually invisible in modern societies. Few parents have any idea about what polio, measles, or a meningococcal infection would mean for their child. Against the background of a very low incidence of these diseases and a concurrent high vaccination rate that results in group immunity, forgoing vaccination might even be considered a rational choice—at least from a self-interested individualistic perspective.

Seeing modern vaccine refusers as fully rational fact-driven deciders, however, is questionable. What unites modern vaccine critics more generally is their view that vaccines might be more dangerous than the diseases they aim to prevent. They actively dispute medical evidence—mostly, in general, "mainstream" biomedical and epidemiological science—and question the ways in which governments provide and promote large-scale vaccination programs. They overestimate the risks of vaccines, and their counterarguments are often fueled by elements of a metaphysical worldview that emphasizes "naturalness" or the purity of the body: they see vaccination, for example, as injecting a human body with a "foreign" substance that is unnatural and thus contaminates the purity of themselves or their newborn child. Their views find support in conspiracy theories on social media, such as the belief that pharmaceutical companies and governments are covering up information about vaccines being unsafe or ineffective. These communications can easily affect people's intention to be vaccinated (Jolley & Douglas, 2014). Parents are encouraged to do their own research (on the internet) and to form their own judgment instead of trusting what governments and physicians say. Doing one's own research is seen to make sense because of alleged biases in scientific research: mainstream science cannot be trusted because it is funded by a pharmaceutical industry that just wants to sell as many vaccines as possible. In these ways, vaccine critics are sowing the seeds of doubt about government-led immunization programs. By appealing to generic concerns about risks, financial interests, and government paternalism, these groups have a much stronger "outreach" and influence than the religious opponents of vaccination.[3]

Mark Navin explains that many parents hook on to this movement after having become disappointed with mainstream medicine or after having felt that their concerns were not taken seriously (Navin, 2016, pp. 21–56). They turn their back on regular health care, seek health providers who will not challenge their beliefs, and sometimes form or join *alternative communities of knowers* (Nyhan et al., 2014). These are explicitly antipaternalistic and anti-authoritarian communities that provide ample space for sidelined voices, including self-identified *parent-researchers* who primarily employ web-based research. Moreover, these communities emphatically endorse democratic norms for allocating epistemic authority:

> Democratization movements and the advent of the Internet have changed the environment around vaccines from top-down expert-to-consumer (vertical) communication towards non-hierarchical, dialogue-based (horizontal) communication, through which the public increasingly questions recommendations of experts and public institutions on the basis of their own, often web-based, research. (Larson et al., 2011, p. 528)

Inspired by these movements, some parents may reject or delay some or all vaccinations for their child, while others will just forgo those vaccines that aim to prevent what they consider to be "innocent diseases"—mumps, varicella, measles, whooping cough—and only protect their child against diseases they consider very dangerous—like diphtheria and polio. The anti-vaccination movement not only is "successful" in persuading people to actively refuse immunizations for their child but also encourages vaccine hesitancy, uncertainty, and doubt among other parents, prompting them to at least postpone vaccinations, request separate vaccines rather than a combination vaccine like MMR, and avoid more than one shot at a time. During the COVID-19 pandemic, when debates about immunization became even more polarized, these strategies were also employed to raise doubts about the novel pandemic vaccines.

3.4 Epistemic Controversies

Even though vaccine criticism is as old as vaccination itself, the current wave of antivaccination sentiment seems to be more intense than earlier resistance and is more capable of attracting the attention of parents still on the fence.[4] Wakefield's MMR *vaccine-causes-autism* claim has propelled a new wave of vaccine critique. A second cause of the upsurge is that the internet and new social media platforms like Facebook and Twitter have offered vaccine critics an unprecedented opportunity to diffuse their message to a much wider audience. How can we understand these phenomena? In this section, we argue that modern vaccine criticism and resistance may be considered symptoms of a broader individualism and of erosion of trust in collective institutions.

When large-scale routine immunizations against poliomyelitis, diphtheria, and other diseases were introduced, this was mostly heralded as a decisive strategy against horrible disease outbreaks. Their success in preventing epidemics and reducing morbidity and mortality was remarkable. Moreover, they arrived at a time when there was strong collective trust in medical authorities and (governmental) public health institutions. People generally seemed to endorse a social contract–like agreement: everyone participated in vaccination programs so that everyone was protected.

However, over time, the collective optimism about the benefits of vaccination slowly evaporated. The urgent public health aim of fighting infectious diseases, quite paradoxically, lost its status and visibility as the devastating effects of these diseases faded from the collective memory. This development coincided with a second, more general social phenomenon of an emerging individualism in the Western world. The collectivist spirit that had sparked the trust in and success of vaccination programs in the early sixties and seventies gradually became overshadowed by a more individualistic assessment of vaccination. As large outbreaks of infectious diseases became less common or even remained absent in high-income countries, people's attention shifted from the importance of protection against epidemics to the (alleged) risks of vaccinations.

Nowadays, a substantial number of worried parents may not be reassured by knowing that the MMR vaccine is effective in protecting against disease and contributes to herd immunity and that, on a population level, the health benefits of vaccination clearly outweigh potential adverse reactions. Instead, such parents are more interested in the question of whether the MMR vaccine is safe for *their own child*. Childhood vaccination programs aiming to preserve herd immunity ultimately lead to a trade-off. Thanks to these programs, individual children are immune, society is safer, and immunocompromised persons and newborn babies are indirectly protected. If a robust group-level protection has been established, it may appear as if vaccination for one's own child is not urgent: they are already protected indirectly. As a result, the attention of many parents has shifted from concerns about disease outbreaks to the risks associated with vaccination.

It may be attractive for proponents of vaccination to reduce vaccine denialism to irrational and antiscientific beliefs. After all, there is overwhelming scientific evidence in support of modern vaccination programs;

population benefits far exceed harmful side effects. However, Goldenberg and other *science, technology, and society* scholars emphasize that public questioning of vaccines in the twenty-first century cannot merely be understood in terms of an antiscience ideology or a misunderstanding of the science (Goldenberg, 2016; Koerth-Baker, 2016). They argue that part of the vaccine criticism and hesitance can be explained by the unilateral focus of scientists and public health authorities on population-level benefits, which largely misses the individual-oriented concerns of parents. This implies, they suggest, that government should not jadedly and repetitively rehearse the importance of herd immunity but instead should engage with parents' arguments about what is best for *their child*.[5] This does not imply that governments must accept every objection to vaccination without scrutiny. But it does require a reorientation of the way governmental agencies communicate the importance of vaccination, not only in terms of a collective focus on public health but also in terms of the best interests of the child involved.

Although Goldenberg and other scholars have a valid point here, governments cannot avoid acknowledging that individualized perspectives will result in a collective-action problem: on an individual basis, for the parents of any child living in a context of herd immunity, it might even be rational to forgo vaccination. At the same time, accepting these individualized perspectives at face value is ultimately self-defeating as a policy. If more parents avoid the minimal risk that vaccinating their child entails, fewer children are vaccinated, which increases the likelihood of an outbreak. Vaccination, as well as yielding a private good—the protection of the individual—also contributes to the public good of herd immunity. The collective-action character of herd immunity has long been unnoticed, because group protection simply flowed from large numbers of parents who had their children vaccinated for private, not collective, reasons primarily concerned with the health of their offspring. Herd immunity achieved in this way is only a positive externality that results from many private choices. The trend of diminishing vaccination rates in the first decades of this millennium shows that herd immunity does not have a stable basis: it is in fact a contingent positive externality of individual choices that can evaporate over time.

It is only to be expected that parents would reconsider their vaccine hesitancy if risks of measles outbreaks reappear. But it would be cynical for a government to wait until outbreaks recur to regenerate public awareness of the dangers of vaccine-preventable childhood diseases—doing so would sacrifice the health or even the lives of children. Moreover, one cannot expect that most vaccine-hesitant people will change their mind if the risks are less remote: vaccine refusal has also been common during the COVID-19 pandemic. Many people had doubts about the severity of the disease and assumed that vaccination was unnecessary. Luckily, a large majority of people do participate in regular national programs, and vaccine denialism remains only a minority view.[6] At the same time, coverage of childhood immunization has decreased throughout the past few decades in many countries. Antivaccination groups appear to have been successful in influencing parents who are uncertain but feel that they are responsible for making their own choice about vaccination. As mentioned previously, they herald the idea that each parent should do their own research and form their own judgment about the benefits and burdens of vaccination. Social media enable laypersons to exchange stories, rumors, and experiences with other parents. They can even explore the vast collection of biomedical scientific literature. Parents who are interested and concerned about side effects of vaccines will easily find sources that are in line with those concerns: personal anecdotes of parents whose children became severely ill just days after being immunized or scientific reports about side effects. Antivaccination groups are eager to bring all such experiences, alleged experiences, anecdotes, and scientific reports together and then invite other parents to read it, which is framed as "doing their own research" and "making up their own mind."

Developing a well-informed position in this debate is, however, less straightforward than these groups make it seem. Scientific research into vaccination has produced a robust body of knowledge that has been generated over a long period of time and is based on research in various disciplines. Yet the conclusions drawn from this research are not offered on a silver platter in a straightforward way. Instead, they are to be derived from many articles that are scattered across a large range of scientific journals. To genuinely appreciate this body of knowledge, one needs to have a comprehensive view of the evidence. One cannot conclude on the basis of one or two (or even dozens of) scientific articles that vaccines do or do not work or that they are harmful. It is easy to find scientific publications that note harmful effects. It is even easier to find publications that emphasize the benefits. But a good scientific judgment must be based on a review of the entire body of knowledge in the field.

It is already hard for professionals to keep up with the literature, so it is virtually impossible for laypeople to develop an overview of the scientific field. By suggesting that laypeople can "do their own research" and by emphasizing that everyone is able to determine what the risks and benefits of vaccines are, vaccine critics suggest they take a neutral stance ("respecting autonomy"). But in fact, they undermine public confidence in science, in biomedical scientists and other experts, and in public health programs.

Given the fact that most citizens are not experts in this field, participating in national immunization programs presupposes a certain level of public trust in vaccinations and in the government agencies and professionals that implement them. This implies that citizens have to accept medical expertise and competence and that they defer to specialists the weighing of risks and benefits concerning issues beyond their knowledge (Sorrell, 2007). Maintaining that trust, or gaining it if it is not already there, is a difficult task. We discuss the problem of trust in more depth in chapter 9.

Even if, from a medical or public health point of view, immunization is the preferred (if not obviously best) choice, no one can deny the reality of epistemic and ethical disputes about deciding whether or not to participate. Whether people object to vaccination for religious reasons, because of a particular "nature-centered" worldview, because they are more concerned about the risks than about the benefits of immunization, or because they simply do not trust mainstream scientists or government officials, such objections cannot just be pushed aside by appealing to a scientific and professional consensus. This is not only because a blunt rejection of concerns might easily reinforce distrust in health authorities. Much more importantly, in a liberal-democratic society, the plurality of worldviews should be acknowledged and therefore the concerns and choices of citizens must be taken seriously—also if these choices are not in line with scientifically grounded medical recommendations.

3.5 Taking Opposition Seriously

A core characteristic of liberal democracies is that the freedom and autonomy of citizens are respected and considered cornerstones of the liberal-democratic tradition itself. Respect for personal autonomy implies that citizens have the freedom to form and revise their conceptions of the good life and to organize their lives accordingly. This acknowledges the Kantian normative axiom that all human beings have equal dignity, which implies that no person or group is allowed to dominate, suppress, or otherwise impose their will on others. It also recognizes the value of a plurality of different and sometimes conflicting ideas of the good life and, indeed, that a good society is one where people with different worldviews—religious or secular—can coexist peacefully. In the long run, a good quality of life is best attained if individuals are free, in a negative as well as a positive sense, to make their own choices (and mistakes) in life.

At the same time, liberty is inevitably limited: if all persons deserve respect, then each person's liberty is necessarily constrained by the liberty of others. As John Rawls's first principle of justice formulates, each citizen in a liberal-democratic state "is to have an equal right to the most extensive total system of equal basic liberties that is *compatible with a similar system of liberty for all*" (Rawls, 1971/1999, p. 266, emphasis added). Indeed, one of the key questions of liberal-democratic political philosophy concerns the legitimate constraints on individual freedom and whether there are further grounds for interfering with individual freedom apart from liberty itself.

This implies that government should provide space in which citizens can make up their own mind about vaccination and that it takes those persons who express objections to vaccination seriously. This has important implications for our discussion on vaccination hesitancy and refusal. Vaccine-hesitant citizens can have various reasons why they reject vaccination. Many of them refer to a fundamental gut feeling about "autonomy" or "noninterference" and the belief that decisions concerning immunization of themselves and their child are *their* choices, which government should not interfere in. Even though these are fundamental and legitimate *moral* convictions, they need to be unpacked and translated into relevant *legal* rights before they can be invoked as a shield against interference by government. This implies that the predominantly moral concepts of autonomy and noninterference must be "disaggregated" (Laborde, 2017) into specific legal claims that are acknowledged by courts and have to be realized to a certain threshold to guarantee autonomy.

In the context of immunization policies, respect for personal autonomy can be unpacked and linked to specific legal rights by appealing to the notions of *bodily integrity, freedom of thought and religion,* and a *right to family life and parental autonomy.* In the remaining sections of this chapter, we aim to formulate the argument for respecting objections to immunization in the strongest possible sense. More precisely, we argue that a democratic government cannot set objections aside just because they have good medical and public health reasons for aiming at high immunization rates. Chapters 4 through 7 discuss the limitations of this argument in the case of childhood vaccination; chapter 8 discusses the limitations of coercive vaccination of adults. In those chapters, we explain how, even though the objections are taken seriously, government is sometimes allowed and required to introduce liberty-limiting measures to promote immunization.

3.6 Bodily Integrity

The freedom to decide what others can(not) do with one's body or the freedom to resist others to intervene in one's body is arguably a fundamental right of every person. This right is sometimes linked to the idea of self-ownership (Locke, 1988; Nozick, 1974). Moreover, if we assume that human beings have a right to privacy, then the bodily sphere seems to be "private" in the most basic sense. Any idea concerning personal autonomy and privacy is devoid of content if it does not contain a right to control interventions in and on one's body.[7] For that reason, it is now generally accepted that a medical intervention should not be imposed on an individual without their *informed consent*. A competent person's well-considered refusal of medical treatment is not an absolute barrier for physicians starting or continuing therapy but certainly one that is almost unsurpassable. Health care professionals may have good reasons to question a person's choice to refuse medically beneficial treatment, but if it appears that the patient's refusal is a well-informed, well-considered, and voluntary choice, they will, rightly, abide by it. This is not only in line with a basic idea about respect for autonomy; normally, an individual will also be the best judge of their own best interests, which are broader than health alone. Obtaining informed consent for medical interventions is therefore firmly embedded in medical ethics and medical law, but that does not imply that it is merely a matter of professional obligation within health care: the grounds for requiring informed consent for medical treatment apply to other persons, institutions, and governmental agencies too. The Dutch constitution expresses this explicitly as the inviolability of the human body. According to article 8 of the European Convention of Human Rights (ECHR) jurisprudence, the right to private life also includes "the physical and moral integrity of the person."[8] The European Court of Human Rights concluded that "even minor medical treatment against the patient's will must be regarded as an interference with the right to respect for private life."[9]

These fundamental human rights protecting bodily integrity are not absolute, and often legal provisions specify under what conditions the state is allowed to make exceptions. In liberal democracies, those exceptions are quite limited. Some examples are taking blood or saliva samples from convicted criminals for DNA analysis or doing alcohol-level tests on car drivers. It might be argued that mandatory seatbelt wearing is also a restriction of the right to bodily integrity; this measure is common and presumably widely accepted in all jurisdictions. The clearest cases in which "bodily integrity" is at stake, however, concern interventions or actions that intervene *in* the body or cause physical pain—without proper consent. Vaccination certainly falls into that category, which is why it is a major barrier for public health authorities that want to require citizens to be vaccinated. Whether there is a sufficient ethical ground to justify compulsory vaccination programs, and therefore to see vaccination as a legitimate exception to the right to autonomy and bodily Integrity, remains to be seen.

Arguably, the rights to autonomy and bodily integrity are at their strongest when a competent person is refusing medical treatment for themselves. Autonomy and bodily integrity presuppose a unity of mind and body: *I determine what happens to my body*. Therefore, another person, including a medical doctor, is not allowed to do things to a person without their informed consent. This implies that the right to the integrity of the body presupposes a competent person who can autonomously accept or refuse an intervention. This will be an important argument in the discussion of vaccination for adults, for example, in the context of COVID-19, and we will discuss this in chapter 8.

However, in the context of childhood vaccination, this argument is less straightforward (Pierik & Verweij, 2022). Most programs target children who are not yet competent decision makers, so the authority to consent to medical treatment usually falls to their parents or legal guardian, and they are supposed to make such decisions based on the best interest of the child. It is not immediately obvious, however, that a medical intervention on a child without *the parent's* consent would be an infringement of *the child's* bodily integrity. Indeed, as we argue in chapter 5, when parents and the state disagree about what is in the best interests of the child, it is not always the case that parents have the final say. The American Academy of Pediatrics therefore also favors the language of "parental permission" instead of the much more stringent concept of parental *consent* (Katz et al., 2016).

To assess the validity and strength of the argument about the bodily integrity of the child, we must assess how the concept can be understood in this context. One possible reading is to take bodily integrity literally, as "wholeness," where surgery or other medical procedures interfere in the body and thus violate its integrity. This reading is untenable, though, as it would imply that many, if not all, medical interventions violate bodily integrity, even if parents had consented to treatment. It is, often, however, the other way around: medical interventions, if appropriate, aim to *preserve* bodily integrity where it is threatened due to an injury or disease. Successful therapeutic interventions heal persons and their bodies; they do not violate them. Preventive treatments like vaccines also preserve and protect bodily "wholeness" by making the body immune to certain infections. Of course, medical treatment can also have harmful side effects, and thus even well-intended vaccinations may occasionally threaten bodily health and integrity—but whether the preventive intervention can be considered *ex ante* as a violation of bodily integrity amounts to an assessment of the benefits and risks of the intervention for the child. In other words, arguments about bodily integrity ultimately amount to determining what is in the best interests of the child. Given the fact that young children are incapable of making such decisions themselves, and for reasons we discuss later (section 3.8 and chapter 5), it is the parents who are in principle designated as the guardians of their child and authorized to make choices in their best interests. Note, however, that by reducing the argument about bodily integrity to an assessment of a child's best interests, the rhetorical force of the idea of bodily integrity itself evaporates.

Yet this view, that all body- or health-preserving interventions necessarily respect integrity, presupposes a concept of bodily integrity that is fully naturalistic or biomedical and disregards the *normative* meaning of integrity. Acknowledging the normative dimensions implies that a person's bodily integrity is only at stake when their bodily sphere is invaded *by someone who is not authorized to do so*.[10] In our view, there is always only one person who without any doubt can be considered having this authority, and that is the person whose body it is. Indeed, the normative force of the right to bodily integrity is this direct link: it is *your* right that it is *you* who determines what happens to *your* body. If the person whose body is interfered with cannot make the decision themselves to authorize the intervention, then the force of the argument deflates. When an authorization of a medical intervention must be made by a guardian—either parents or the state—there is no inherent argument *from the perspective of bodily integrity* that explains why parents are *ipso facto* better situated to make this decision than the state. As we argue in chapter 5, parental prerogative is the most plausible starting point of this discussion, but it is not an absolute principle.

We have argued that in principle, the right to bodily integrity is a strong argument against governments imposing biomedical interventions on citizens. However, the right to bodily integrity is not absolute; it can still be overruled on other legal grounds, as happens in the case of mandatory alcohol tests, so it remains to be seen whether the right to bodily integrity is strong enough to overrule compulsory or mandatory immunization. In chapter 8, we elaborate further on this delicate balance between the individual right to bodily integrity and possible overriding concerns in the context of COVID-19 vaccination programs for adults.

Second, we have shown that the strength of appeals to the right to bodily integrity is highly questionable if it concerns childhood immunization. Parents cannot claim they are the sole guardian of their child's bodily integrity, and, moreover, it may even be argued that safe and effective immunization, even if imposed against the will of parents, preserves, rather than violates, the child's bodily integrity. This theme is elaborated further in chapter 5.

3.7   Freedom of Thought, Conscience, and Religion or Belief

A second fundamental ground for taking objections to immunization seriously is to respect liberty of thought and religion. The rights to freedom of thought, conscience, and religion or belief have been laid down in various international conventions, including the International Covenant on Civil and Political Rights (ICCPR, art. 18) and the ECHR (art. 9). These rights protect not only specific beliefs but also people's choices and desires to live in line with their religious beliefs or worldview or, as the ICCPR describes it, "to manifest his religion or belief in worship, observance, practice and teaching." Freedom of thought is one of the most basic prerequisites of a liberal democracy, sometimes even seen as "the basic and distinctive 'first freedom' in the liberal political order" (Pierik, 2015, p. 254).

It goes without saying that the concerns of some religious groups about immunization (e.g., that it interferes with divine providence) and the ensuing objections to vaccination policies fall under the scope of these rights. Enforcing immunization would obviously violate the liberty of members of these groups to live according to their religion. The same applies to comprehensive anthroposophist worldviews that include metaphysical ideas implying that childhood diseases are important steps in a child's development. Moreover, the fundamental right at stake is not limited to religions or comprehensive worldviews; other convictions also deserve protection. The European Court does not require that substantial criteria are met for a person's conviction to qualify as a "belief" in the sense of the freedom of religion or belief. Instead, it simply requires that the conviction must display "a certain level of cogency, seriousness, cohesion, and importance."[11] Recently, however, the court concluded that the mere disbelief of facts about vaccination, without it being substantively embedded in a broader religious of philosophical worldview, cannot count as a coherent personal philosophy of life that is sufficient for protection under article 9 ("Vavřička," 2021, ¶29, ¶335). Still, many parents embed their fear of side effects in a more comprehensive worldview, and therefore they may well be justified in arguing that their freedom of thought and religion are at stake. This brief discussion makes it clear that governments and public health professionals have very strong reasons to take objections against vaccination seriously and cannot just push them aside via coercive policies.

There are however, two caveats. First of all, as explained above, the protection of liberty and basic rights and respect for autonomy are fundamental moral and legal principles, but they cannot be absolute, specifically not when the health interests of other individuals, or of society at large, are at stake. This proviso is made explicit in the second section of article 9 of the European Convention:

> Freedom to manifest one's religion or beliefs shall be subject only to such limitations as are prescribed by law and are necessary in a democratic society in the interests of public safety, for the protection of public order, health or morals, or for the protection of the rights and freedoms of others.

In more general terms, this proviso was famously put forward by John Stuart Mill in what is now called the harm principle: freedom can be legitimately constrained to prevent harm to others. The principle is relevant for vaccination programs to the extent that immunization not only protects the vaccinee but in most cases also contributes to the protection of other persons, for example, those who cannot be vaccinated. In the following chapters, we explore whether the case for vaccination is strong enough to justify setting limits on liberty.

The second caveat, which only applies in the context of childhood vaccination, is even more fundamental. It is questionable whether freedom of thought, conscience, and the religion of parents also protect choices for their children. Adults have rights to freedom of religion, and hence the right to refuse vaccination because of their religion or worldview, but do such rights give them authority to decide for or against vaccination of their children? This issue is taken up in the following section. We argue that there is a strong moral and legal basis for parental prerogative in matters of preventive and curative medical treatment of their children. But as we show in later chapters, once again, such rights are certainly not absolute.

3.8 Respect for Parental Autonomy

So far, we have established that there are two strong yet not absolute ethical grounds, bodily integrity and freedom of conscience, for respecting and therefore not pushing aside people's refusal of and hesitance about vaccinations. These grounds are also backed by legal frameworks such as the European Convention of Human Rights and jurisprudence in the European Court. Both fundamental rights can be seen as protecting individual autonomy: a person's right to govern their own life and live according to their own conception of the good. What still needs to be established more clearly is whether and why such autonomy would also include the authority to make decisions for one's young children—does personal autonomy also imply *parental autonomy*?

Justifications for respecting parental autonomy can be consequentialist and nonconsequentialist. Consequentialist arguments will see parental autonomy as a means to promote other values, such as the well-being of the child and the family. Given that almost all parents care about their children and desire the best for them, and that they are in a very good position to assess their child's needs in specific situations, it is reasonable to assume that, normally, they will make choices that are in their child's best interests. The government might set certain standards (e.g., certain general requirements for a good education), but individual parents will be much better situated to decide which educational approach fits their child best. The same may apply to specific medical choices.

The second consequentialist ground for respecting parental autonomy is that parents may have to weigh conflicting interests and demands of children and other family members. Choices that are perfect for one child (e.g., a special school that is relatively far from home, a camping holiday full of physical activities, saving more money for college) might be disadvantageous for her brother. Parents are well situated to decide trade-offs in a way that is best for the family as a whole. Fostering a safe, private sphere of family life can also contribute to establishing affective and caring relations between all family members and raising children in a way that means they learn to care for one another (Diekema, 2004, p. 244).

A first nonconsequentialist argument for granting parents authority to make decisions about what is best for their children is that parental *autonomy* is a necessary condition for parental *responsibility*. The idea that parents have special duties of care toward their children is only viable if they are also able to act and decide accordingly. Acting for the sake of duty presupposes freedom to do so; without freedom (even freedom to fail), responsibility is empty and meaningless.

The second nonconsequentialist argument revolves around the idea that for many parents and parents-to-be, their individual autonomy cannot easily be separated from parental autonomy. Giving birth to a child, caring for them, seeing them grow up, and educating them to become a person with a life of their own are all major elements of what constitutes *their own life* and can be decisive regarding what it is to live a good life. The choices that mothers and fathers make for their children thus also determine and shape their own lives. Moreover, for a person who takes their own view of the good life and their own values seriously, and who also deeply cares for their children, it would be a major restriction of freedom if they were not allowed to raise their children in line with those values or to expose their children to them and inspire their children to live according to those values.

The caveat we mentioned previously applies here as well: fundamental rights are not without limits. Yes, there are strong grounds for parental autonomy that gives parents authority to make pedagogic, educational, medical, and other important decisions for their young children. Parents have the freedom and responsibility to make decisions in their child's best interests as determined by the parents themselves—this is what parental autonomy is all about. However, their conception of *best* interests may sometimes conflict with what, from a higher-order perspective, is considered the child's most *basic* interests. In chapter 5, we explore this distinction between basic and best interests in depth, and we argue that a liberal-democratic government has a responsibility to secure basic interests of children and that this implies limits to parental autonomy.

This idea of parental autonomy is often framed in terms of a right to family life, as laid down in, for example, article 8 of the European Convention. But the Convention also makes clear that this right is not absolute. The second paragraph of article 8 asserts that statutes enacted by national parliaments can limit this freedom when it "is necessary in a democratic society . . . for the protection of health or morals, or for the protection of the rights and freedoms of others." This has implications for the right of parents to refuse vaccination for their children. Indeed, in *Vavřička*, the European Court decided that the parental prerogative not to vaccinate can legitimately be constrained if a coercive vaccination policy is necessary to protect children and the public against vaccine-preventable diseases ("Vavřička," 2021, ¶284–288).

3.9   Fundamental Rights and Their Limitations

In this chapter, we presented some of the main reasons specific groups have for rejecting vaccination for themselves or their children. In most countries, such strong objections are held only by relatively small minorities; most people do accept vaccinations without hesitation. At the same time, there are many who are at least hesitant or otherwise have doubts about vaccines, and these groups offer fertile ground for vocal antivaccination groups to share and spread their deep objections. This is a matter of concern for governments, public health authorities, and medical professionals. In a pluralist democratic state, the government cannot simply suppress deviant views or restrict the freedom of citizens to determine their own lives and, to some extent, those of their children. Hence, the conflicting ethical and legal considerations require further analysis to find answers that are reasonable and proportionate.

It should be emphasized that in both liberal-democratic political philosophy and liberal-democratic law, fundamental rights are paramount, and they can only be restricted under very explicit conditions. But this also implies that rights to the freedom of thought, conscience, and religion or belief cannot be absolute; in specific circumstances, they are subject to restrictions that are "in accordance with law" and "necessary in a democratic society to protect the rights and freedoms of others" (ECHR, art. 9). In a similar vein, the right to family life and the resulting right to parental autonomy can be restricted by the state when this is necessary to protect the interests of the child.

In the legal domain, the principle of proportionality is widely employed to determine whether an infringement of basic rights is justified. The central idea is that a government's interference in citizens' freedom must not be disproportional, given the goal the law seeks to achieve, which already presupposes implicitly that the law as such is justified. The principle is usually employed in a four-pronged test (Alexy, 2014, pp. 52–54; Brems & Lavrysen, 2015, p. 141; Klatt & Meister, 2012, pp. 8–10; Rivers, 2014). Given the circumstances of the case, four elements must be analyzed.

First, there must be a legitimate purpose for a measure that infringes the fundamental right. This condition is much more stringent than just the idea that the measure should have a goal that is beneficial. Not every societal benefit justifies what is at stake here: an infringement of liberty. If the state is to restrict individual liberty, the purpose should at least be an important element of the core tasks of the government. Some constitutions or conventions even specify what grounds are considered legitimate purposes for such an infringement and under what conditions these apply. For example, article 9 of the European Convention of Human Rights holds that "freedom to manifest one's religion or beliefs shall be subject only to such limitations as are prescribed by law and are necessary in a democratic society in the interests of public safety, for the protection of public order, health or morals, or for the protection of the rights and freedoms of others."

Second, the measure must be suitable for achieving the purpose, and this can include a requirement that there is (scientific) evidence to show that the measure will do so. Obviously, if the measure is futile, the purpose cannot justify the restriction of fundamental freedoms. The second part of the condition—the ideal that the measure is *evidence based*—raises an important question: what level of evidence can be gained beforehand about the effectiveness of a policy measure? Even though intrusive policies need to be based on the best available scientific evidence, decisions will often also involve some level of uncertainty about effectiveness, as the various policies drafted in response to the COVID-19 pandemic have made perfectly clear.

Third, the measure, as well as being suitable for achieving the purpose, must also be *necessary* to achieve the purpose. That is, there should not be an alternative, less onerous measure that could achieve the purpose equally well. This principle is known as the *principle of subsidiarity*, or the principle of least restrictive alternative or least intrusive means.

Fourth and finally, the measure must be reasonable in view of the competing interests of the citizens at stake. This last element of the test of proportionality is certainly not the least important: it involves weighing the competing claims and values at stake. Is the infringement of certain fundamental liberties (respect for autonomy, freedom of thought and religion, right to family life) proportionate given the purpose and necessity of maintaining herd immunity?

This form of legal reasoning that revolves around the principle of proportionality seems to be more dominant in the European legal tradition (Kumm, 2007, p. 154), but "it is also an increasingly common feature of rights-based judicial review in most other constitutional democracies worldwide" (Dixon, 2017, p. 2199). Indeed, various authors have argued that, contrary to the widespread idea that the proportionality approach is quite alien to the US constitutional tradition, there are more similarities than dissimilarities and that the proportionality approach quite closely resembles a "strict scrutiny approach" (Jackson, 2015, pp. 3104–3120; Sweet & Mathews, 2019, pp. 96–162). In addition, the idea of a proportional weighing of values and principles is also central in medical-ethical and legal-philosophical discussions. Therefore, we endorse it as an important method for the analysis in this book.

The first condition is paramount and principled. If there is no legitimate purpose for a measure that infringes the fundamental right, the measure can never be justified. The latter three conditions concern weighting factors where all kinds of contextual arguments play a role. Jointly, these conditions typically structure legal judgments of, for example, the European Court of Human Rights. This court has the final say in cases where citizens contest the restriction of the individual exercise of a fundamental right by a state party to the Convention.

In the next two chapters, we first discuss the principled basis for state coercion. Can the use of force to compel people to get vaccinated be legitimate at all? What specific arguments apply if it is about parents refusing vaccination on behalf of their child? From chapter 6 onward, we explore in detail whether and how immunization policies can restrict liberty in proportionate ways.

4 A Principled Argument for Liberty-Limiting Vaccination Policies

In chapter 2, we argued that the state has a compelling interest in preventing (major) outbreaks of infectious diseases. By far the most effective way in which such outbreaks can be precluded is through the establishment and maintenance of robust herd immunity in cases where this is possible, and the only way such collective protection can be maintained is through mass vaccination. A disease like measles used to be endemic in most societies, and this led to regular outbreaks, but thanks to immunization programs, it became a rather abstract and remote risk, at least in high-income countries.[1] However, measles outbreaks such as the 2015 Disneyland outbreak in California, those in various European countries in 2018, and the 2019 outbreak in the city of New York have provided parents and the public with renewed firsthand experience of the reality of (the threat of) these diseases and their harmful impact. When herd immunity is hard to attain, or when it can no longer be taken for granted because of an emerging vaccine hesitancy, the question arises whether coercive policies are justified.[2]

In this chapter, we develop a principled argument for liberty-limiting vaccination policies by exploring the implications of John Stuart Mill's "harm principle." This principle offers the strongest possible justification for liberty-limiting vaccination policies: constraining freedom of individuals is justified if it is necessary to prevent harm to others. There are different ways in which a choice to forgo vaccination (for oneself or, more often, for one's child) can be harmful or at least impose a risk to others. First, an unvaccinated person can encounter the disease, fall ill, and, subsequently, infect and thus directly harm other persons. Second, even if an unvaccinated individual does not directly cause severe disease in another person, they still add to the risk of a pathogen transmitting from person to person. The aggregated effect of the many individual decisions not to vaccinate is that the disease is more likely to spread and that the collective good of herd protection is undermined in society. Herd immunity not only protects the health of vulnerable groups (as discussed in section 2.2) but also prevents societal disruption and damage caused by outbreaks. We argue that the second application of the harm principle—which appeals to the protection of the public good of herd immunity—does at least offer a principled ground for policies that sets limits to the freedom to forgo vaccination for oneself or for one's child. There is also a third possible route for how the harm principle is relevant to immunization: parents' choice to resist having their children immunized might be considered a matter of harm *to the children themselves.* We discuss this specific argument more in detail in chapter 5.

The public good of herd immunity is often also referred to in a different strand of ethical arguments, namely, that vaccination refusal amounts to *unfair freeriding* (see, e.g., Buttenheim & Asch, 2013; van den Hoven, 2013). We explore this argument in section 4.4 but show that the argument of fairness is not fully successful.

4.1 John Stuart Mill's Harm Principle

In chapter 2, we presented several types of nonvoluntary immunization policies. Mandatory, compulsory, and forced vaccination policies all involve clear limits on the freedom of choice of citizens. The most solid reason for restricting individual liberty is the prevention of harm to others—as eloquently argued by John Stuart Mill in his essay *On Liberty* (1991). Mill analyzes the nature and limits of the power that collective bodies like the state can legitimately exercise over the individual. He argues that

> the sole end for which mankind are warranted, individually or collectively, in interfering with the liberty of action of any of their number, is self-protection. That the only purpose for which power can be rightfully exercised over any member of a civilized community, against his will, is to prevent harm to others. His own good, either physical or moral, is not a sufficient warrant. (Mill, 1991, p. 14)

Mill embraced the liberal idea that a government, or society at large, has no legitimate power to force individuals to behave and live the lives that others (government, religious leaders, a majority) deem best for them. Such paternalism, "either physical or moral," cannot be justified. Mill argues that everyone should have absolute freedom as long as it concerns "self-regarding" choices—that is, choices that only affect their own interests. The state does have a central role, however, in regulating behavior that can harm the interests *of others*.

This so-called harm principle is one of the cornerstones of the contemporary liberal-democratic tradition in legal and political philosophy. Its strength can be explained by pointing out how it captures the idea that liberty must be constrained within a society. After all, how one person uses their freedom will often affect the freedom and opportunities of others. If liberty had no limits—that is, if everyone were free to do as they wished irrespective of how their actions would affect the lives of others—in the end, no one's freedom could be ensured. There would be nothing to prevent others from taking "the freedom" to steal your property, to endanger your life or health, or to coerce you to do or believe what they wanted you to. Of course, most people would not do these things, but in a democratic society, government should protect the freedom of all citizens to shape their own lives. To protect each person's freedom, the freedom of all must, to a certain extent, be limited. This element of the harm principle—that prevention of harm to others is in principle a good ground for setting limits on freedom—is something that every democratic perspective must endorse. One does not have to be as straightforward a liberal as John Stuart Mill to endorse this position. Every democrat, whether egalitarian, libertarian, communitarian, or socialist, must agree that the state is justified in limiting everyone's freedom if this is necessary to prevent harm to others. The antipaternalist strand in Mill's philosophy, or, more broadly, his assumption that prevention of harm to others is *the only ground* for coercion, will be much more controversial. For our purposes, we can focus on the uncontroversial part of the harm principle: curtailing people's freedom to prevent them from harming others is, in principle, justified.[3]

Of course, this is not about any minor harm or inconvenience. If it comes to state coercion, Mill employs a rather strict conceptualization of harm: "interests, which, either by express legal provision or by tacit understanding, ought to be considered as rights" (Mill, 1991, p. 83). Acts of individuals that are hurtful or lack due consideration for the welfare of others but that do not violate any of their constituted rights may not be punished by law, only by opinion (Mill, 1991, p. 83). Arguably, protection against severe infectious diseases does fit within such a restricted conceptualization of harm, and this opens the door for seeing a choice to avoid vaccination as harmful. Mill's principle concerns the prevention not only of intentional (or malevolent) harm but also of actions that unintentionally affect the basic interests of others, which is specifically relevant for our discussion. In the case of a contagious disease, persons can unknowingly—hence unintentionally—contract a disease, transmit it to others, and amplify an outbreak.

Governments have compelling reasons to prevent that from happening. The harm principle implies that the state is justified in limiting the freedom or autonomy of citizens when this is necessary to prevent persons infecting others and thus spreading disease. Some contagious diseases can spread through the air, via coughing and sneezing, and others are spread via direct skin contact or exposure to body fluids or materials (blood, feces, etc.). Immunization is arguably the most effective route to avoid getting infected and spreading a disease to others; a well-considered decision to forgo freely available vaccinations might therefore be considered a case of allowing the possibility that one will harm others. In the following sections, we discuss two ways in which such a choice could be harmful and thus be considered a ground for the government to curtail individual liberty: it may result in direct infection and therefore the harm of others, and it may undermine and harm the public good of herd protection. In chapter 5, we explore a different way of seeing nonvaccination as harmful: as parents' choice to disregard their own child's basic interests.

4.2   Vaccination Refusal as Causing Direct Harm to Others

Consider the following two examples, taken from recent newspaper articles. In an article in the *New York Times* in 2015, Tamar Lewin presented the case of Rhett Krawitt, a then six-year-old boy with leukemia. After four years of chemotherapy, the boy was vulnerable to infections and therefore could not be vaccinated (Lewin, 2015). Because his health was so fragile, it was essential that as many people as possible around him were vaccinated, because being infected with a disease such as measles could have been fatal for him. But his parents were struggling with the fact that many children at his school, including some in his classroom, had not been vaccinated because parents had "philosophical" objections against immunization. What if one of these unvaccinated classmates infected him with the disease? Shouldn't schools or the government prevent such infections—for example, by denying unvaccinated children access to schools?

Or consider this example from March 2014 in the Netherlands. A child whose parents had decided not to participate in the vaccination program was infected with measles, and before the symptoms of the disease became manifest, she attended a day care center and therefore exposed several other children there to the pathogen. As a result, three babies fell ill. Micha, a six-month-old baby—too young to be vaccinated himself—suffered from severe complications, had to be treated in intensive care for a few days, and almost died. In an interview with the Dutch newspaper *de Volkskrant*, Micha's mother said, "They took a gamble with the health of my child. I cannot stop them from deciding not to vaccinate their children. But don't send your unvaccinated children to a nursery in which young babies are crawling around who, because of their young age have not yet been vaccinated" (Effting, 2014). Such cross-infections can especially occur in child day care centers, because unprotected younger babies (the first MMR vaccination is only administered when a child is twelve to fifteen months old) often share facilities with children up to four years old. Older toddlers are usually more adventurous and mobile than younger ones and therefore have a much bigger chance of contracting and spreading disease. Micha was harmed by being infected, and this could have been precluded easily and safely if the older child—the vector—had been vaccinated. The moral judgment of the baby's mother about the parents of the older child is understandable. Normally, we do expect parents to take care that their own children do not harm or pose a risk to the health of other children.

These cases illustrate why a common defense cited by vaccination refusers does not hold. This defense consists of an argument that no one can complain that vaccine refusers cause a risk—after all, people who do endorse immunization will be protected because they have chosen to be vaccinated. Vaccine skeptics use this argument to reduce vaccination to a self-regarding choice, and this challenges our appeal to the harm principle. Their argument, however, does not hold because many children are, like Micha, too young to be vaccinated and thus vulnerable to infections. Other persons, like Rhett, are highly vulnerable and cannot be immunized, or they have been immunized as a child but have become vulnerable due to immune-compromising diseases or the frailties that come with old age. Forgoing vaccination is not "merely" a self-regarding choice; it does impose a risk and can indeed cause harm, not just to oneself but to others as well. Of course, that does not imply that such a choice is malevolent; the harm is not intended, but it remains a consequence of a choice.

Jessica Flanigan makes an analogy with other choices that have unintended harmful effects. She compares vaccine refusal with celebratory gunfire: people are not entitled to impose deadly risks on others, and this applies to both cases (Flanigan, 2014). By firing guns in the air while celebrating Independence Day in the US, patriot gunmen risk other people getting hit by bullets that fall back down to the ground. She argues that even though this risk may be remote, it is not a reason to conclude that a prohibition of such gunfire is unjustified. In several states, celebratory gunfire is a misdemeanor that is punishable even if the gunfire does not harm anyone. If the analogy holds, we have a ground to prohibit vaccine refusal as this also creates a risk that an individual—or their child—is causing serious harm to others.

A weakness in Flanigan's position is that it suggests that any action that involves increased risk of injury to others might be a candidate for being prohibited. Lots of things we do, and should have the right to do, increase the risk of harm to others. Biking around on a Sunday afternoon increases the risk of harm to pedestrians, and leaving a backyard pool unsupervised increases the risks that the children who live next door sneak in for a swim and drown. It is not so much about whether our acts increase the risk of harm to others but whether this increased risk can be publicly justified as part of a socially beneficial scheme (Brennan, 2018). Is the small extra risk that nonvaccination generates justifiable? One argument that says that it is suggests that fundamental rights are at stake, such as the freedom of religion of nonvaccinating citizens, and that compulsory vaccination might violate bodily integrity. This requires the government to balance the social interest of countering the risk of nonvaccination with the recognition of the fundamental rights of nonvaccinators, which we do in the upcoming chapters.

Another possible problem in Flanigan's analogy is that the wrongness of celebratory gunfire involves a wrong *act* and the wrongness of nonvaccination is a matter of *inaction* or *omission*. John Stuart Mill, however, explicitly also ranks certain inactions as falling within the scope of the harm principle.[4]

> A person may cause evil to others not only by his actions but by his inaction, and in either case he is justly accountable to them for the injury. The latter case, it is true, requires a much more cautious exercise of compulsion than the former. To make any one answerable for doing evil to others, is the rule; to make him

answerable for not preventing evil, is, comparatively speaking, the exception. Yet there are many cases clear enough and grave enough to justify that exception. (Mill, 1991, pp. 15–16)

Mill considers this to be specifically relevant in the context of collective endeavors undertaken for mutual benefit: every member who receives the protection of society owes a return for that benefit and "the fact of living in society renders it indispensable that each should be bound to observe a certain line of conduct towards the rest." This implies not only not harming the relevant interests of others but also "bearing his share (to be fixed on some equitable principle) of the labors and sacrifices incurred for defending the society or its members from injury and molestation" (Mill, 1991, p. 83). Vaccination programs can be considered exactly what Mill describes here: collective, socially beneficial schemes that offer protection to society at large.

The upshot of this first application of the harm principle is that although it is possible to see forgoing vaccination as a matter of *creating a risk of direct harm*, the seriousness of that risk needs to be evaluated in the context of the broader societal benefits that vaccination programs offer.

4.3 Compelling Persons to Contribute to Herd Immunity

Mill not only discusses the implications of the harm principle for choices that may lead to infecting and thus directly harming other individuals but also considers the idea that people can make choices that are harmful in an indirect way, insofar as these undermine certain societal goals. More specifically, he invokes the principle as a possible basis for compelling members of society to contribute to collective projects that benefit all. The harm principle thus also allows enforcing a person to do

positive acts for the benefit of others, which he may rightfully be compelled to perform, such as to give evidence in a court of justice; to bear his fair share in the common defence, or in any other joint work necessary to the interest of the society of which he enjoys the protection. (Mill, 1991, p. 15)

We will argue that mass immunization aiming at herd protection is such a joint work necessary to the interest of society and that the state is justified to limit individual freedom on those grounds.

Our argument proceeds in two steps. We first reformulate the various benefits of herd protection and explain how these constitute a public good. Subsequently, we discuss separately the case where vaccine coverage is still far too low to achieve robust group protection and the case where such group-level protection is already secured. We claim that achieving and maintaining group-level protection against a very serious disease that is threatening public health and societal life is in the shared interest of everyone in that population. As argued before, this shared interest is closely linked to one of the core functions of the state. Vaccine refusal is not merely a failure to contribute; it also undermines the collective endeavor to protect an important public good, and therefore we see it as causing harm to all.

4.3.1 The Public Good of Herd Protection

The group-level protection that comes with herd immunity surfaces if sufficient people have become immune, either through experiencing the disease or through vaccination. The importance of establishing and maintaining group protection against serious diseases is obvious. First of all, it offers specific protection for children like Micha (section 4.2) who are too young to have completed their immunization schedule, for immunocompromised patients like Rhett, and for persons whose immune system has responded insufficiently to vaccination. Second, group-level protection reduces the risk of outbreaks; outbreaks will inhibit interpersonal contact, either through infectious disease control measures (isolation, quarantine, closing of childcare centers or schools, etc., as happened in spring 2020 during the COVID-19 outbreak) or through fear of infection. Indeed, during an outbreak of a disease, fear of infection may spread more rapidly than the infectious disease itself, and this has an impact on social life even if the outbreak remains contained. In these ways, the prevention of outbreaks is clearly important.

Herd protection thus brings multiple benefits. Interestingly, many of these benefits are open to all—to people who do opt for vaccination and also to those who do not vaccinate themselves or their children. Herd protection is a *public good* because it has the following features (Dawson, 2007). First, the good cannot be produced by an individual alone but requires a cooperative scheme. To produce the outcome, general though not necessarily universal compliance is required, and it also involves an ongoing activity—it is not a one-off event. This is clearly the case with group protection: we need collective immunization programs to achieve a coverage required for herd immunity, and group protection can only be sustained if almost all children receive their shots.

Second, once it is produced, the public good is *nondivisible*—the benefits cannot be divided within a group; it is *nonrivalrous*—one person's use of it does not limit its use by others; and, most important, it is *nonexcludable*—it is impossible to exclude individuals from benefiting from this good. This implies that there is a similarity and a difference between those who cooperate in the scheme and those who don't. The similarity is that noncooperators have equal access to the benefits of the cooperative effort. As explained above, herd immunity protects the health of many persons and the well-functioning of society that is relevant to everyone, vaccine enthusiasts, hesitant parents, and straightforward vaccine refusers alike. The difference is that only cooperative persons contribute to the provision of the public good, while vaccine refusers do not.

Such public goods are usually indispensable for society because they involve the provision of services that are necessary for societies to flourish, such as public education, protection against crime, general societal infrastructures, or military defense. At the same time, they are vulnerable since they can only be generated by collective action, and given that benefits will be available to collaborators as well as noncollaborators, there is a risk that some people will seek to refrain from doing their share. According to Mill, failure to do one's fair share in such a cooperative effort is causing harm to society (and thus other citizens within society), which can be a reason for the state to act and enforce or compel citizens to contribute.[5]

One of the best examples of an indispensable public good is the protection against floods in regions that are close to the sea or to rivers. For instance, in the Netherlands, almost one-third of all the populated land is below sea level, and for centuries, local societies have built dikes and created polders to expand livable areas, and they have maintained those polders by draining out the water. Obviously, maintaining the dikes and other water-related works to prevent flooding is a necessary condition for public safety and thus for societal life, and thereby an essential public good. Throughout history, the building of dikes and other water-related works to protect against floods has been realized as a collaborative effort, which, on a larger scale, would have been impossible without a government that steered activities and, if necessary, also enforced people to contribute through physical labor or taxes.

Protection against infectious diseases through the establishment of group-level protection is another example of such a public good. Indeed, if we consider it a case of "joint work necessary to the interest of the society of which he enjoys the protection," Mill's harm principle can support curtailing individual freedom to refuse vaccination. Let us unpack this argument in two parts, which apply to two different contexts.[6]

4.3.2 Striving toward Group-Level Protection against an Immediate or Imminent Threat

The COVID-19 pandemic has provided the world with firsthand experience of the impact of both a novel and dangerous infectious disease and the harsh social distancing measures that are necessary to control it. The pandemic has shown not only that many people fall ill and die but also that hospitals become overwhelmed with patients requiring life-saving medical care. The measures that must be taken in response to a pandemic can bring social life to a standstill: schools, workplaces, and restaurants are closed; public transportation is limited; and people may not be allowed to leave their homes and must work from home and homeschool their children. There may be various ways to overcome such a disaster, but if a disease can be combatted by immunization, and if such a vaccine becomes available, collective vaccination seems to be the best possible and most effective route to contain and stop the epidemic. As in many other vaccination programs, policies that promote the adoption of a new vaccine serve two aims: to protect individuals against the risks of symptomatic disease and to inhibit or stop the spread of infection within the population. Circumstances might be such that achieving herd protection is even considered indispensable to containing the epidemic for a long time and to be able to lift all infection control measures that brought social life to a grinding halt. If it is indeed a novel virus, no one is protected, and the focus cannot be limited to childhood vaccination. In chapter 8, we use the COVID-19 pandemic case in more depth to illustrate the ethical discussions surrounding the vaccination of adults. For now, we focus on the following general question: can the harm principle be invoked as an argument for setting limits to freedom of choice if herd protection has not yet been attained?

First of all, it is clear that if achieving a high vaccination rate leads to group-level protection, it will benefit each and every one of us—those who are still vulnerable but also those who are already immune. We all have an interest in common: as members of the public, we are vulnerable, if not to the infection itself, then at least for the disruptive effects of outbreaks and the necessary control measures. It will be important to achieve and maintain a situation in which quarantine, lockdowns, and other measures are not necessary anymore and can be lifted.

Given the stakes that all of us have in stopping the epidemic, it is reasonable to claim that all of us are harmed if some groups actively refuse vaccination and thus obstruct or inhibit the objective of group-level protection. Their refusal is on par with refusal to follow necessary social distancing measures to slow down or contain an epidemic. It could be that complying with the measures and, for example, undergoing tests and quarantine if a test is positive is, for some, a reasonable alternative to vaccination. But vaccination refusal may still inhibit a collective attempt to achieve herd protection. Therefore, governments can appeal to the harm principle to justify liberty-limiting policies that compel citizens to accept vaccination. This is in line with the core tasks of government: to protect its population against major threats now and in the future, to ensure the prerequisites for an open society, and to protect the basic interests of adults and young citizens who, for medical reasons, cannot protect themselves. If a democratic government initiates such a program but then sees the objective of group protection endangered by the noncompliance of some groups, vaccination refusal can be considered as harming others or, more specifically, as harming an interest that every person has in their capacity as a member of the public.[7] Whether or not a mandatory or compulsory policy is actually justified and proportionate will depend on a myriad of factors. Yet in a case like this, the harm principle offers a clear basis for justifying the infringement of liberty for the sake of protecting society via herd immunity.[8]

4.3.3   Maintaining the Public Good of Robust Herd Protection

Interestingly, the public good of herd protection mostly emerges as a positive externality of individual choices of people who primarily seek to protect themselves or their own child. This dimension makes vaccination different from many other collective goods, and we discuss that in more depth in section 4.4. This predominantly private incentive to vaccinate means that vaccination programs have a much better chance of establishing collective protection on a voluntary basis than, for example, the collective endeavor of building dikes or the joint defense of military services. Ideally, this incentive would be so common and strong that robust herd immunity would be established and maintained voluntarily, and governments would have no reason to use force and set limits on individual freedom. There would still be a principled ground for coercion—because the harm principle would be applicable—but enforcing it would be unnecessary. Mill acknowledges that

> there are often good reasons for not holding him to the responsibility . . . either because it is a kind of case in which he is on the whole likely to act better, when left to his own discretion, than when controlled in any way in which society have it in their power to control him. (Mill, 1991, p. 16)

Unfortunately, in the past few decades, people have become increasingly hesitant or skeptical toward vaccination: the private benefits of immunization appear insufficiently visible or persuasive for them, and indeed a significant number—though still a small minority—forgo vaccination. As a result, vaccination coverage against diseases like measles and pertussis is not optimal, and even if group-level protection is established, it is not as robust as one would hope. More and more national governments have considered and sometimes adopted mandatory programs to counter this tendency.

This leaves us, however, with an important question. So far, we have argued that the harm principle offers a reason for states to restrict the freedom of individuals (notably parents) to refuse vaccination offered by basic programs, because this means that the state ensures collective protection against outbreaks of serious infectious diseases. But is coercion necessary if, as it happens, most people comply anyway and if the number of voluntary vaccinations is sufficient to achieve group-level protection? It is indeed a central, if not defining, feature of public goods that they require general but not necessarily universal compliance. If herd protection is established through general compliance because most people collaborate voluntarily, it seems as if an individual's refusal to contribute cannot be phrased in terms of harm to others. After all, the noncooperation of a still small minority will make little to no difference to the successful maintenance of the public good and thus can hardly be considered harmful to others. Does this imply that our appeal to the harm principle is not convincing if herd immunity is established?

This is a specific version of a common problem in discussing collective harms (Cripps, 2011; Kagan, 2011; Nefsky, 2012, 2019; Polkamp, 2019). If one individual's actions as such do not seem to be much of a difference to the harm that might occur—but would occur only if many acted like them—how can *their* choice be considered a case of harm to others? If this is a ground to restrict their freedom, it seems as if they are penalized for what others are doing. How can that be justified?

For several reasons, we believe this skepticism about collective harm is misplaced, and certainly so in the case of vaccination policies. First, we endorse Elisabeth Cripps's general analysis of collective harm. If individuals contribute to collective harms like climate change or outbreaks of infectious diseases, those persons should not be held responsible for their individual choice. The individuals taken together are *collectively* responsible in the sense of being responsible as a putative group who *jointly* cause harm. As Cripps argues, curtailment of their individual freedom is prima facie legitimate when the duties imposed on the individuals are fairly allocated as part of a collective endeavor to prevent that harm (Cripps, 2011), and that is what occurs in a mandatory vaccination program.[9]

Second, even in circumstances of herd immunity, the risk of harm is real. There is no reason to assume that voluntary programs will guarantee sufficient group-level protection in the longer run. Few countries (with or without mandatory programs) have been successful in establishing and maintaining complete herd immunity—which in the case of measles would require approximately 95 percent of the population to be vaccinated—certainly not since the modern vaccination hesitance has gained ground. Even if hesitant and actively refusing parents are still a minority, their number is large enough to obstruct the establishment of such a high coverage. As a result, outbreaks can and do occur, as witnessed, for example, between 2016 and 2019 in Ukraine, Italy, and the city of New York—even outbreaks that were severe enough to disrupt societal life. This offers a justification for the state to initiate vaccine mandates.

Third, one should not underestimate how refusals undermine collective protection even if the protection is already in place. Noncollaboration is not merely a matter of "not doing one's part" by contributing to a public good; it involves leaving a weakness in the collective protection in place. A good analogy is citizens building a wall together to protect the city against enemies. If you don't do your part by putting some bricks in the wall, the other citizens will have a larger burden and will probably do "your part" as well. Yet collective vaccination is different: the protective "wall" here consists of all persons who are vaccinated (or otherwise immune), so if you choose not to be vaccinated, you create a weakness in the collective protection that cannot be compensated for by others. When the protective "wall" is complete, there will still be a hole at the spot where you were supposed to lay your bricks.[10] In this way, each and every failure to collaborate generates a weakness in the protection of public health and, as such, undermines the collective endeavor at large.

David Lyons argues that if not contributing to important public goods cannot independently be characterized as harmful to other individuals, the contribution of everyone is still required because the collective endeavor supports a social practice that prevents significant harm (Lyons, 1979). This argument also applies to immunization. Although vaccination remains the norm, there is—and there will probably remain—a vocal minority of hesitant parents that remains doubtful about the necessity and safety of vaccination for their children. Such hesitance may be criticized from a scientific point of view, but in a society in which diseases like measles and polio have become uncommon, and in which rumors about real or alleged side effects of vaccination easily spread via social media, some hesitance will probably be inevitable. Many of these parents will comply with immunization but will remain susceptible to the concerns that antivaccination groups or other hesitant parents put forward. Moreover, if they see others getting away with just "opting out," with no clear negative consequences, this will make them wonder why they should comply; it facilitates seeing opting out as a reasonable and legitimate option and thus nudges them to forgo immunization as well. In these ways, individual vaccination refusals constitute a collective harm; they undermine the collective endeavor toward the public good of group protection, the prevention of outbreaks, and possibly the (remote yet not impossible) global objective of eradicating diseases like polio and measles.

A related argument is given by Alberto Giubilini (2019, pp. 44–46), who claims that, as a society, and maybe even globally, we have a collective responsibility to prevent dangerous infectious diseases by, where possible, establishing and maintaining herd immunity. Seeing herd immunity not only as a desirable public good and collective endeavor but as something that people collectively *have a moral duty to* establish offers additional support to our analysis. Our argument, however, goes one step further: it is not just that people have a moral duty to contribute to herd protection; we argue that vaccination refusals undermine policies that are part of the state's central tasks: to maintain group-level protection against infectious diseases. Citizens have a right to such protection, and those rights are impeded—though indirectly—by people who deliberately opt out of a well-established vaccination program.

In short, vaccine refusal undermines an important collective endeavor that is meant to prevent harm, and in that sense, it can be seen as falling within the scope of the harm principle. Moreover, if vaccination refusal becomes more common, the group-level protection may fall apart, leading to more disease outbreaks and thus more widespread harm—which would us bring back to the scenario of the previous subsection.

4.3.4 Nonvoluntary Vaccination Policies: A Moral and a Legal Perspective

We conclude that vaccination refusal can be considered to fit within the scope of the harm principle and that within a liberal democracy, there is ground for restricting the individual liberty not to be vaccinated. It may be difficult to argue that the state is justified in compelling individuals to accept vaccination for themselves or their children as a matter of preventing direct harm to concrete others, but nonvaccination is certainly a matter of harm to others as it undermines the collective endeavor necessary to establish and maintain herd immunity. Mill's harm principle thus serves as a justification for the government to make vaccinations against serious diseases mandatory or compulsory. This claim is also in line with several legal cases and democratically accepted policies. A landmark court case in the US is *Jacobson v. Massachusetts*, in which the Supreme Court allowed a compulsory immunization campaign after the 1901–1903 smallpox outbreak in Boston. According to the court,

> The liberty secured by the constitution of the United States to every person within its jurisdiction does not import an absolute right in each person to be, at all times and in all circumstances, wholly freed from restraint. There are manifold restraints to which every person is necessarily subject for the common good.

The Court established that the state "may impose reasonable regulations to ensure the public health and safety, even if such regulations infringe individuals' personal liberty."[11] The goods of public health and safety require collective action and collaboration, and state power may be necessary to ensure such cooperation. In more recent times, the European Court of Human Rights has in various decisions allowed domestic authorities to mandate vaccination. In *Solomakhin v. Ukraine* (2012) and *Boffa and others v. San Marino*

(1998), the court ruled that limits can be set to the right to private and family life (art. 8 of the European Convention of Human Rights) and to the freedom of thought, conscience, and religion (art. 9) in order to protect the health and the rights of others.[12] Most recently, in *Vavřička* (2021), the court ruled that the mandatory Czech immunization policy is indeed a limitation of parental prerogative (art. 8), but it is a justified limitation given that it serves a legitimate purpose:

> The objective of the relevant legislation is to protect against diseases which may pose a serious risk to health. This refers both to those who receive the vaccinations concerned as well as those who cannot be vaccinated and are thus in a state of vulnerability, relying on the attainment of a high level of vaccination within society at large for protection against the contagious diseases in question. This objective corresponds to the aims of the protection of health and the protection of the rights of others, recognised by Article 8. ("Vavřička," 2021, p. 60, ¶ 272)

The court thus emphasized not only the protection of the individual vaccinee but also the indirect protection of vulnerable persons via herd protection (we discuss this issue further in chapter 5). Finally, recent government decisions to implement or tighten mandatory vaccinations against measles in, for example, Italy, France, California, and New York City, have also survived democratic and legal scrutiny (Camilleri, 2019, p. 247).

The justification in terms of the harm principle is most clear in contexts where herd immunity has not yet been established in a robust way, but we have also explained that there is a ground for compulsion in cases where herd immunity is more solid. In the latter case, the justification may be less strong because there is some room for refusal of vaccination. In the next chapters, we analyze how this can play a role in designing proportionate policies. First, though, we explore a different route that can be taken, which could offer additional support for nonvoluntary vaccination when coverage is already more than sufficient. This is the argument that in such a case, if refusal is not clearly harmful, it would still be *unfair*.

4.4   Freeriding: Is Fairness an Additional Argument for Vaccine Mandates?

Enjoying the benefits that arise from a collectively produced good without doing one's share toward its production may not only be seen as morally problematic because it harms society's collective endeavor to maintain a public good. It can also be considered morally repulsive for other reasons. Enjoying the benefits of a joint enterprise without contributing to the collective project is often labeled "freeriding." The term can be used descriptively, just to describe that type of behavior, but it is often used as an evaluative or even derogatory concept, which implies that such behavior is considered intrinsically wrong. The wrongness of freeriding might offer an additional route toward liberty-limiting government intervention to enforce collaboration. The argument would then be one of fairness: it is unfair to reap the benefits of a joint enterprise without sharing in the burdens that are needed to produce the good. More in general, democratic governments should see to it that burdens and benefits of policies are distributed in a fair and equitable way. The principle of fairness is applied to vaccination in Alberto Giubilini's justification for compulsory vaccination (2019). In the following subsections, [13] we present his justification and further explore the argument about the unfairness of freeriding. We reject the argument of fairness, however, because it does not take into account the fact that herd immunity is a very peculiar type of public good—one that supervenes on private goods.

4.4.1   Vaccination Refusal as Unfair Freeriding?

For Alberto Giubilini, the starting point is that citizens *collectively* have an *obligation* to contribute to important public goods (2019). This is an appealing idea, certainly for a problem like global warming. The challenges that climate change creates for the current and future generations are enormous, and given that global warming is clearly the result of the CO_2 emissions that are caused by our modern way of living, humanity should take responsibility for preventing further emissions and mitigating the effects of climate change. It makes sense to see this responsibility as a collective responsibility as we are creating the problem together and also because attempts by individual persons to mitigate climate change are futile unless they are embedded in a concerted action with many other people.

In a similar vein, contagious diseases spread from human to human, which involves all of us as causal links. Collective protection also requires concerted efforts, and this can be seen as supporting a collective responsibility to achieve herd immunity. The question is, though, how such joint obligation relates to the duties of each individual citizen. One could argue that individuals who refrain from doing their part are harming others, as we have done in the previous sections. Giubilini, however, focuses on how the benefits and burdens of the collective obligation are distributed:

> Thus, the collective obligation to realize herd immunity generates a certain amount of "burdens": a certain number of individuals will have to be vaccinated. I call vaccination "a burden" in this context because some people are opposed to it and because vaccination does involve some small inconvenience (possible temporary pain of the injection, having to pay a visit to the doctor, potentially a financial cost, minor risk of some side effects, etc.). . . . In any case, the relevant question, for our purposes, is the question as to how such burdens should be distributed among individuals who form the collective with the moral obligation to realize herd immunity. It is safe to assume that such burdens should be distributed fairly, to the extent that we think that fairness is an important value that needs to be taken into account when distributing any kind of burden involved in the realization of important public goods. Thus, fairness demands that each individual does whatever she reasonably can in order to contribute to the fulfilment of the collective or shared obligation, regardless of the actual impact any individual action would have on the realization of the collective outcome. (Giubilini, 2019, pp. 50–51)

In other words, the principle of fairness requires that any individual who can contribute to herd immunity and who can bear the (small) burdens, that is, persons without medical exemptions, should do their fair share regarding the fulfillment of the collective obligation. This is in line with Mill's argument that the harm principle can involve compelling people to *do their fair share* and accept the burdens that this involves in the collective projects from which they benefit as well. We have already argued that the harm principle does justify compelling people to contribute to the joint project of herd immunity because it prevents harm, but we did this without discussing the "fair share" element in more detail. We can now see how fairness sets two constraints. First, the harm principle cannot—as a matter of fairness—demand more of individuals than that they should do their fair share. In this sense, it sets a constraint on what can be required. Arguably, as far as contributions to herd immunity are concerned, the only thing that most people can do is to have themselves or their children vaccinated— so in that sense, everybody's contribution is equal. In other contexts, for example, concerning our joint obligation to reduce CO_2 emissions, it is possible that your "fair share" is much larger than mine, if only because you emit much higher levels of greenhouse gases than I do or because, due to your wealth, you are in a much better position to make more sustainable but also more expensive choices.

Second, fairness also implies that each of us should *at least* accept and bear our fair share of the burdens of establishing herd immunity. Of course, these burdens are only minor inconveniences and remote side effects, but it still makes sense to distribute burdens and benefits in an equitable way. If there are various ways to divide and distribute benefits and if the stakes of a collective project are very high—that is, if the benefits but also the burdens are significant for most people involved—we might need to discuss in more detail what an equitable distribution involves. Should individuals who are worst off in some sense be exempted from sharing in the burdens? Or should those who contribute most to the collective risk (i.e., spread of infection) bear a larger share? In vaccination programs, there is only one way to contribute, which is to be vaccinated, and the burdens are minimal. In this context, a relatively simple understanding of fairness may initially be sufficient: reaping the benefits of a collective project but refusing to contribute to it and share the burdens of it is not fair.

The advantage of this line of argument, compared to our own public goods account of the harm principle, is that it may offer a justification of compulsory vaccination that does not lose any of its strength in a context of robust herd immunity. As explained earlier in this chapter, the harm prevention justification for mandatory immunization is less strong in such a context: nonvaccination can still be considered harmful as it impedes the collective undertaking, but the harmful effects on public health might well be negligible. If we can make a case that nonvaccination is also *unfair*, though, this argument applies regardless of whether herd immunity is at risk or whether such group protection is robustly established. Even if 99 percent of citizens voluntarily comply and accept the burdens of immunization, the remaining 1 percent who refuse are still acting unfairly: they enjoy the benefits but refuse to contribute.

What is at stake here is, of course, that vaccination refusal in a context of herd protection amounts to freeriding. The central moral problem of freeriding is not just that it may undermine the realization of the public good but that some people *take a free ride* when others all share in the burdens of producing the good. The wrongness has to do with how people take advantage of others without reciprocating, and this may imply an unfair distribution of burdens and benefits. The claim about the unfairness of freeriding regarding a jointly produced public good is difficult to resist—and this is not different in the case of vaccination. The intuitively most objectionable case of freeriding is encouraged by Robert Sears, a US antivaccination celebrity also known as "Dr. Bob," who is blatantly honest in his advice to nonvaccinating parents: "I also warn them not to share their fears with their neighbors, because if too many people avoid the MMR vaccine, we'll likely see the disease increase significantly" (Sears, 2007, pp. 96–97, as quoted in Navin, 2016, p. 143). This advice, deleted in the second edition of his book (Sears, 2011), clearly reflects a deliberate intention to freeride on the cooperative practices of other people. How can it be fair to seek to benefit from herd immunity as much as anyone else but not to contribute a fair share—especially where we jointly have an obligation to achieve such a public good? Of course, many vaccination refusers are not that explicit about their intention to freeride. And in the case of parents who object to vaccination on anthroposophist grounds and who would *prefer* their children to be exposed to measles (see section 3.2), it is questionable whether their rejection of vaccines amounts to freeriding at all. Bradley and Navin (2021) argue that vaccine refusal is hardly ever motivated by the idea of profiting from other people's choices to participate in collective schemes, and therefore they hold that vaccine refusal is not to be considered freeriding at all. However, we deem parents who refuse immunization to be free riders, because they consider the risk for their child too high given the remote benefits. These parents do endorse the fact that the chance their child will be infected is relatively small. But that fact is a result of successful collective vaccination, that is, the cooperation of most other parents in immunization schemes. So they are having a "free ride" even though few of them will perceive it in that way. The question, then, is whether such a choice is unfair.

Before analyzing this stance about the unfairness of vaccination freeriding, let us briefly take a closer look at the concept of fairness itself and try to grasp what makes unfair practices wrong. This is not an easy task, because "fairness" is such a basic and intuitively appealing idea that it is hard to pin it down in straightforward terms. Few authors have been working on the concept of fairness as closely as John Rawls did, but even he seems unable to offer a precise definition. This is probably the best we can get:

> The concept of fairness . . . relates to right dealing between persons who are cooperating with or competing against one another, as when one speaks of fair games, fair competition, and fair bargains. The question of fairness arises when free persons, who have no authority over one another, are engaging in a joint activity and amongst themselves settling or acknowledging the rules which define it, and which determine the respective shares in its benefits and burdens. A practice will strike the parties as fair if none feels that, by participating in it, they or any of the

others are taken advantage of, or forced to give in to claims which they do not regard as legitimate. (Rawls, 1958, p. 178)

Fairness only makes sense in a context in which free and reasonable people acknowledge certain rules as legitimately guiding how they should relate to one another. A fair distribution of burdens and benefits of social cooperation is, then, one that is determined by general principles that all can agree with. If certain beneficial goods can only be made available to anyone if (almost) all contribute to its creation—as in a public good—and if such contribution comes with not insignificant costs, then it is reasonable for people to reject free riders: individuals who deliberately reap the benefits of the collective endeavor without contributing and thus take advantage of those who do contribute.

This shows a lack of respect for others as free and equal individuals and also for the importance of having mutually beneficial practices and rules. Moreover, by reaping, hence accepting, those benefits, others can reasonably claim that they voluntarily commit themselves to the societal scheme and thereby to an obligation to do their fair share. It is like freely deciding to engage in a particular societal practice or play a game: doing so commits one to follow the rules of the practice or game as well. In Rawls's view on public goods, accepting the benefits is one of the conditions for seeing cooperative action as something that is morally required as a matter of fairness (Rawls, 1971, pp. 111–112).

Whether or not accepting the benefits is a necessary condition for seeing freeriding as unfair has been subject of philosophical debate. Garret Cullity argues that under specific conditions (collaboration results in a net benefit, the obligation to collaborate is generalizable, and refusers have no legitimate moral objection to the scheme), freeriding is always unfair. Deliberately accepting the benefits or appreciating the public good at stake is not among those conditions. Cullity's analysis is applied to immunization by Mariëtte van den Hoven, who infers that all vaccination refusers who benefit from herd immunity engage in unfair freeriding, simply because they choose not to do their fair share in the collective scheme (van den Hoven, 2013).

Whether or not one follows Rawls's more restricted account of unfairness or Cullity's expanded fairness principle, it seems clear that Robert Sears's advice as quoted above amounts to unfair freeriding. The same applies to vaccine refusers who see the risk of immunization as outweighing the remote benefits, although less visible. As we argued in response to Bradley and Navin's suggestions, these parents can only consider the benefits as remote given the fact that most people are immunized and thus have contributed to herd protection. In this way, refusers do assume the benefits of the public good.

More debate is possible when we focus on religious refusers and anthroposophists. On the one hand, they could respond that they avoid Rawls's criterion as they do not voluntarily accept the "benefits" of group immunity; these are imposed on them, and they would rather avoid them. On the other hand, they could claim that a vaccination scheme—at least *from their perspective*—does not result in a net benefit at all, thereby resisting the first of Cullity's conditions for unfair freeriding. Moreover, religious refusers could appeal to their freedom of religion that is infringed, thus claiming to have a legitimate objection to the scheme, which implies that Cullity's third condition does not apply either. Although we cannot fully agree with these responses, we will not elaborate this discussion.[14] We do not need to because, ultimately, the argument that vaccination refusal is unfair fails for other reasons: as we show in the next subsection, vaccination freeriding does *not* result in an unfair distribution of burdens and benefits. The principle of fairness therefore does not offer additional support (at least not one that is independent of the harm principle) for setting limits to freedom of choice.

4.4.2 The Peculiar Public Good of Herd Immunity: Freeriding Is Not Unfair

Central to our understanding of the wrongness of freeriding is that the distribution of benefits and burdens involved in the production of a public good should be fair. This involves, at least, that those benefits are open to all and that the costs are shared equitably. In this section, we argue that the distribution of benefits and costs, especially the costs, that comes with maintaining herd protection is not unfair, even if certain groups do take a free ride. This implies that neither vaccination freeriding nor immunization policies that allow room for freeriding are unfair.

The main reason why vaccination free riding cannot be unfair is that the public good of group-level protection supervenes on the private benefits of everyone who gets vaccinated. In this respect, it differs from many, if not most, other public goods. By definition, a public good can only come about if there is sufficient cooperative action (realized through government policy or more spontaneous collective efforts), and if the good comes about, then everyone benefits: it is nonexcludable. If there is insufficient support, or if the collective effort is otherwise insufficient, the collective good will not come about, and no one will benefit. If a dike along a riverbank has been realized for only 90 percent of the required length, then everyone will have wet feet or worse, and the efforts of the contributors to build the dike will have been completely in vain. Either the dike is fully completed, and it protects everyone, or it is not, and then no one is protected and all the contributions were in vain. In other cases, people will still benefit to some extent, in relation to the proportion of citizens who were willing to cooperate. For example, in a case involving the collective efforts of fishermen to refrain from polluting a lake, if many of them are willing to cooperate, most of the potential pollution will be averted. But here, too, everyone benefits but the burdens are only carried by those who are willing to contribute.

Interestingly, the public good of herd immunity comes about only via individuals who seek and realize personal immunity against infection for themselves. It is unlikely that many individuals opt for vaccination for the sake of contributing to herd immunity: they first and foremost opt for vaccination to protect their child or themselves.[15] This protection comes with some inconveniences and even a very small risk of serious side effects, but generally, people see the individual benefits as by far outweighing the burdens. And if a sufficient number of people have managed to receive protection for themselves or their children, then group protection arises as an "added benefit." Whether or not this added benefit is attained, every vaccinated individual will benefit from their own vaccination anyway—apart from a few individuals for whom the vaccine fails to be effective. If the number of people who participate is insufficient for group protection, almost each vaccinated individual will still be protected and benefit; this is exactly what happens in HPV vaccination campaigns that only target girls and not boys.

Herd protection is an important public good that comes about as a result of many people successfully securing protection for themselves and their children. This is what makes herd immunity a peculiar public good: it is a public good that supervenes on private goods. For each vaccinated person, the attainment of herd protection offers only a minor, perhaps even a negligible, added benefit. However, for society at large, it is significant. Herd immunity protects all children who are too young to be vaccinated and other vulnerable groups such as elderly people or immunocompromised patients. Vaccination refusers also clearly benefit from collective protection even though they do not contribute to the collective effort to achieve herd immunity—hence, they do not share the burdens. But are there any burdens at all for individuals who do contribute to herd immunity? Vaccination offers them individual protection, and herd immunity is an added benefit that comes about, free of charge, if vaccine coverage is sufficient.

Therefore, those who get vaccinated cannot complain that free riders unfairly reap the benefits without sharing in the burdens: from the perspective of vaccinating individuals, there are no burdens at all in producing herd protection. But if herd immunity constitutes a benefit that is open to all, at no cost or no burden, then *the distribution of burdens and benefits cannot be unfair*. This is a remarkable result, especially if one also considers that noncooperators profit much more from the public good of herd protection than collaborators do.[16]

Yet even if the distribution of burdens and benefits cannot be considered unfair, isn't vaccination refusal as such unfair? Maybe it is not about how burdens and benefits are distributed but about the moral character of the choice that defectors make: they don't do what they ought to do—contribute their part of a collective moral obligation, as Giubilini puts it. Although we think there are good reasons to criticize such choices from an ethical perspective, it is less clear how this is, as such, a sufficient ground for constraining their freedom; this is independent, of course, from the conclusion we reached in section 4.3. Vaccination refusal constitutes a collective harm that falls within the scope of the harm principle. The assumption that certain choices are immoral—because of the failure to do what is morally required—is not as such a ground for a curtailment of freedom in a liberal democracy. Although it will be clear that we are making *ethical* judgments about vaccine refusals throughout this book, our primary aim is to discuss the *political* argument concerning how liberal-democratic states should deal with persons who do not voluntarily participate in these programs and thus undermine the collective endeavor of establishing robust collective protection.

To be clear, this does not imply that vaccination freeriding is morally acceptable; it is still wrong because it is morally objectionable as it shows a lack of solidarity with vulnerable persons who depend on herd protection. To put it more strongly, free riders occupy the "protective seat" in the herd that was meant for the most vulnerable persons, and that can rightly be considered morally repulsive.

The conclusion is that even though vaccine refusal can be considered morally objectionable because it involves freeriding on the public good of herd protection, this does not generate a new argument for nonvoluntary policies in addition to those we have already presented in section 4.3. Vaccination freeriding might be morally objectionable, but it is not unfair in a sense that warrants a liberty-limiting policy.

4.5 Conditions for Mandatory or Compulsory Immunization

Let us take stock: in this chapter, we have offered a principled justification for vaccination policies that restrict individual liberties and freedom of choice. Central to our argument is John Stuart Mill's harm principle and, more specifically, the necessity it generates for governments to maintain herd protection. Our argument, which revolves around collective protection and the public good of herd immunity, is not so much an *ethical* argument about interpersonal harms or the moral wrongness of freeriding; instead, it is a *political* argument about rights and collective harms. It starts by asserting that the state has a responsibility to protect people's rights and that robust herd immunity is one of the necessary means for protecting these rights. In this approach, individual vaccination refusal primarily constitutes a *collective* harm, since it undermines the collective endeavor toward group protection.

Individual vaccination is a necessary means for achieving herd immunity, and this justifies state-promoted vaccination through national immunization programs. It can even, in specific circumstances, justify more coercive programs to ensure that members of the political community contribute their fair share to herd protection as a public good in the Millian sense: "a joint work necessary to the interest of the society of which he enjoys the protection."

And the democracy argument kicks in here (Klosko, 1992, pp. 39–51; Simmons, 1979, p. 320). As we have already argued in section 1.9, it is essential for constitutional liberal democracies to strike a fair balance between democratic decision-making and the protection of fundamental rights.[17] Since those who want to establish the public good wish to impose an obligation on the noncooperator and to limit their freedom, they have the burden of proof. They should provide compelling arguments confirming why it is *necessary* to establish the public good, why the cooperation of all is essential in the bringing about of the public good, and why the legal obligations it generates do not *disproportionately* limit the rights and freedoms of those who object (cf. the proportionality test, as presented in section 3.9). The noncooperator is invited to present arguments that oppose these arguments, but there is no *ipso facto* reason why the objector should have the power of a veto within a democracy against the obligation to do one's fair share to bring about an essential public good like the collective protection against (massive) outbreaks of vaccine-preventable diseases.[18] In a liberal democracy, the majority can, in the process of political deliberation and democratic decision-making, be justified in overruling the objection of the minority, as long as the public good to be achieved is considered essential and the infringements of fundamental rights are not disproportional.

But what does that imply in practice? Under what conditions would more coercive policies be justified? What would they look like in the case of childhood vaccination and in the case of vaccination for adults? And what other considerations are relevant? These questions set the agenda for the next chapters. Chapters 5–7 develop the argument for childhood vaccination, and chapter 8 develops the argument for vaccination for adults. Note, however, that our principled basis for mandatory or compulsory vaccination presupposes the following six elements.

First, there is sufficient (scientific) evidence that the vaccines in question are effective and safe. Scientific evidence cannot offer complete certainty, but the evidence is beyond reasonable doubt regarding those vaccinations commonly included in the national immunization programs of the various liberal-democratic states. In extraordinary contexts, it may be reasonable to proceed with compulsory vaccination even if one would have preferred more evidence before doing so—for example, during the outbreak of a novel virus—but these situations would be exceptions.

Second, the vaccines commonly included in national programs offer protection against diseases that are serious on both individual and population levels. Evidence about disease burden may support this, but ultimately this is a value judgment. In this book, we often focus on measles, assuming that the seriousness of this infection is beyond doubt. But in chapter 7, we discuss whether other, less severe diseases or vaccines that do not generate herd immunity can be included in mandatory childhood immunization programs as well.

Third, the infringement of liberty should be in proportion to the harm that is to be prevented. We outlined the principle of proportionality at the end of chapter 3. Judging proportionality involves taking the context of policies into account, and we do so in the next chapters, first focusing on childhood immunization (chapters 5–7) and then on the immunization of adults (chapter 8).

Fourth, the implementation of nonvoluntary policies should not be counterproductive in that it leads to a backlash: societal resistance and distrust that ultimately might lead to a decline in immunization coverage instead of an increase. In section 9.4, we return to the issue of vaccine confidence and how liberty-limiting programs can still be trustworthy.

Fifth, the policies implemented should be the outcome of a democratic process. A legitimate interference with fundamental rights requires political deliberation and democratic decision-making. For that matter, a political debate not only is necessary for the legitimacy of policy but also can contribute to gaining sufficient societal support.

The sixth and final consideration is that governments, when they are considering a coercive policy, should reflect on their *all-things-considered* credibility as a public health authority. Given how important it is that people comply with infection control and other public health measures, public health authorities should be trustworthy. Mandatory or compulsory immunization should not be considered "the" solution to a low vaccination rate if government has so far expected people to pay for vaccination themselves. If limited access to vaccination has led to low compliance, then equitable access should be secured before restrictive policies are considered (Toffolutti et al., 2019).

The harm principle can be invoked not only to prevent indirect collective harm (undermining herd protection). It may also be a ground on which the state can intervene in choices that parents make in the interest of their children. In the next chapter, we discuss the extent to which the state should protect children against the potentially harmful consequences of decisions made by nonvaccinating parents.

5 Basic and Best Interests in Childhood Immunization

In the previous chapter, we offered a principled argument claiming that governments are justified in imposing liberty-limiting vaccination policies when this is necessary to prevent harm to others. Diseases like measles pose a significant threat to public health in general and to the basic interests of vulnerable persons. These are the interests that government should protect by establishing the public health goal of herd immunity. We introduced Mill's harm principle, which offers a basis for justifying liberty-limiting vaccination policies, even if this involves a restriction of such basic rights as freedom of conscience, thought, or religion and the right to family life.

In this and the following two chapters, we answer what this implies for vaccination programs for young children. Should the state intervene in choices that parents make in the interests of their small children who are themselves not in a position to determine their own interests? In this chapter, we translate the more general harm principle into the "harm threshold" to answer why and under which circumstances government is allowed (and required) to interfere in parental prerogative. In chapters 6 and 7, we turn to the more contextual factors that determine which childhood vaccination policies are justified and proportionate in what circumstances.

5.1 Childhood Vaccination: The Focus on the Best Interests of the Child

In chapter 3, we discussed the arguments of science and technology scholars like Maya Goldenberg (2016), who emphasize that the current public questioning of childhood vaccination, in particular vaccination against measles, should be understood in terms of a different assessment of the risk of side effects caused by the MMR vaccination, given that the disease became virtually invisible in affluent countries. If, due to immunization programs, we are confronted less and less with outbreaks of childhood diseases, concerns about the side effects of vaccines come into the limelight more. What if it turned out that your child is the exception that suffers from an extremely rare but severe adverse effect? These authors argue that the current vaccine hesitancy can, at least partly, be explained by the public image of vaccination programs being focused too much on increasing and maintaining the collective good of herd immunity, with too little attention given to parental considerations concerning the potential side effects of vaccination for their child. This implies, they hold, that state agencies should not repetitively rehearse the importance of collective benefits like herd immunity but, instead, should engage much more directly with parents' genuine questions about the risks for their child, both of the disease itself *and* of the vaccination against it.

Indeed, one of the determinants that characterizes the current debate is that parents increasingly require a justification of vaccination policies, and there is an uptick in more "active" parental participation in medical decision-making about their children. This dovetails quite nicely with the "best-interests standard," an approach in medical ethics and law used when making important decisions for persons who are not (yet) competent to make such decisions themselves. Since many of the available vaccinations are given to children in their first two years of life, they are not yet competent to make decisions about their own health. The basic idea is that, while making such a decision, the interests of the person involved should be the ultimate guide. This chapter takes this idea, that vaccination policies must be justified in terms of the interests of the child involved, as the starting point for the analysis. But it raises a fundamental question: if the child's best interests are the most important consideration in vaccination decision-making, who should have the final say when parents disagree with medical professionals or government agencies about how to understand these interests? We argue that state agencies can endorse this idea without also accepting what is usually implicitly embedded in this claim: that parents are the best interpreters of how to understand the interests of their child.

5.2   Best Interests, Basic Interests, and "What Is Best for Children"

Parents increasingly require a justification of vaccination policies in terms of the individual benefits for their child, which is, of course, something that we normally expect parents to do. Inevitably, their judgment will be guided by their own conceptions of a good life and their own assessment of the circumstances. In situations where their child requires medical treatment, they will often depend on the pediatrician's assessment of the situation, and ideally, the pediatrician's medical view and their own judgment concur. From a legal and medical-ethical perspective, both are supposed to act in the best interest of the child, defined by Buchanan and Brock as "acting so as to promote maximally the good (i.e. wellbeing) of the incompetent individual" (Buchanan & Brock, 1989, p. 10).[1] The principle is central in children's law through article 3 of the United Nations Convention on the Rights of the Child (UNCRC), which emphasizes that in all actions concerning children, state agencies must take children's best interests as a *primary consideration*. The UNCRC explicitly focuses on children as separate right bearers because of their dependent position, giving them fewer opportunities to defend their interests themselves. In an elucidation, the Committee on the Rights of the Child writes,

> The expression "primary consideration" means that the child's best interests may not be considered on the same level as all other considerations. This strong position is justified by the special situation of the child: dependency, maturity, legal status and, often, voicelessness. Children have less possibility than adults to make a strong case for their own interests, and those involved in decisions affecting them must be explicitly aware of their interests. If the interests of children are not highlighted, they tend to be overlooked. (Committee on the Rights of the Child, 2013, §37)

If we acknowledge children as separate rights bearers, it becomes clear that "best interests" should be used as an objective standard for evaluating decisions that medical practitioners and parents make as fiduciaries *for* the child. However, in some cases, parents and medical practitioners disagree on whether a child needs a specific medical treatment. Jehovah's Witnesses' refusal to consent to a blood transfusion for their children—for example, in the case of a newborn "rhesus baby"—is widely discussed in the literature (Conti et al., 2018; Wolley, 2005). If medical treatment is necessary in cases of an imminent and severe threat to the health of a child, it is usually considered as being objectively in the best interest of that child. Indeed, in such acute situations, a best interests judgment made by medical practitioners and ultimately enforced by judges in a court is relatively straightforward, even if it is disputed by parents.

However, in the case of preventive treatments like vaccination, the "best interest" standard—understood objectively as "acting so as to promote maximally the good (i.e., wellbeing) of the incompetent individual"—is usually less straightforward as guidance. If a medical decision does not involve a situation of clear and present danger, many other medical and nonmedical considerations may also be relevant in determining what is best for the child. This is especially relevant in discussions about protection against major but relatively infrequently occurring risks. Why should a narrow medical perspective, which seeks to fully eliminate this particular health risk, always prevail in such cases? Indeed, absent imminent threats, it makes sense to pay more attention to a variety of (medical and nonmedical) factors that may affect the child's well-being, and different perspectives or worldviews will then lead to diverging judgments about what is best for the child. This implies that the singular conception of "best interests" is not much help in situations where parents contest nonurgent medical interventions proposed by medical specialists.

In the context of this dispute, we propose to unpack the term "best interests" and examine it as two terms: "what is best for the child," as determined by parents, and "basic interests," which is ultimately a matter of government responsibility. We define the concept of "what is best for the child" as the goals that parents are striving for when they raise their children in line with their idea of the good life. For various reasons, the concept should be understood in an open sense. First, there is a wide variety in how parents conceive these best interests, and the liberal state provides parents much leeway when raising their children in line with their ideas of the good life and transmitting those values to their children. This stems from the parental freedom of thought, conscience, and religion, which itself originates from the liberal idea of tolerance toward various ideas of the good life (see also section 3.7). Second, different children have different personalities. What might be good for one child to stimulate and develop them to their full potential might not be good for another. Since parents know their children best, they are in the best situation to assess their children's character, inclinations, talents, and what each needs to develop their potential.

This concept of "what is best for the child" as determined by parents must be clearly distinguished from "basic interests," for which state agencies have final responsibility.[2] Following John Rawls, we define "basic interests" as those higher-order interests that children have in developing and exercising the basic capacities that are indispensable for growing up into a self-reliant and cooperating citizen in one's society (cf. Rawls, 1971/1999, p. viii). The state should ensure the background conditions and necessary prerequisites that guarantee each child's "open future" (Feinberg, 1980; Millum, 2014). Of course, the concepts "basic interests" and "open future" are contested, can be challenged, and should always be open for democratic contestation of some sort (Shapiro, 1999, p. 85). At the same time, child-rearing unavoidably presupposes certain ideas about what is indispensable in the development toward adulthood and which circumstances undermine this development. Pointing out that these ideas are intrinsically controversial does not undermine their necessity. Basic interests are essential, regardless of a child's individual character, convictions, or ideas of the good life. These include at least (Shapiro, 1999, p. 86):

- access to clean water and healthy nutrition;
- basic medical care, including protection against preventable lethal or disabling diseases;
- the protection of physical and social safety, including the right to grow up in a safe environment in which caring relations can flourish and in which the state does not interfere in family life without a compelling reason;
- basic education, enabling children to grow up into self-reliant citizens that can actively engage in our complex societies.

There is a broad legal consensus in democratic societies about the set of basic interests that the state should guarantee for its young citizens. And in virtually all political communities, this set includes protection against infectious diseases, for example, by means of implementing immunization programs.

In the context of medical decisions, we have replaced the singular notion of "best interests," prevalent in law and medical ethics, by the dual notions of "what is best for the child" and "basic interests." Indeed, despite the dominance of the best-interests parlance in constitutional and international law, it makes more sense to argue that the state only has the ultimate responsibility for a child's *basic interests*. After all, do we really think in the context of all-things-considered policies that a liberal-democratic state, restricted by the requirements of state neutrality, should pursue what maximizes the good of the child? Our dual terminology makes it clear that parents and state agencies share a dual regime structure of authority over children. Their roles are complementary since they have different provinces of legitimate authority over children. The state has the fiduciary responsibility to look after the basic interests of children, and against that background, parents have the fiduciary obligation to make decisions about what is best for their child.[3]

In most cases, most of the time, the two fiduciary authorities work in tandem in complementary ways in the interests of the child. The concept of "basic interests" as just defined is in line with what most parents consider is best for their child. However, since there is no clear-cut division between "what is best" and "basic interests," border disputes may arise where the two fiduciary authorities overlap and conflict. Problems emerge when a parent's views of what is good for their child conflict with one or more dimensions of the political consensus on basic interests. People who endorse one or more of the objections we discussed in chapter 3 seem to have ideas about "best interests" that conflict with what is in their child's basic interest. Some parents still believe that the MMR vaccine causes autism, which gives them reason to consider vaccination harmful and hence not good for their child (Deer, 2011a, 2011b). Others follow Rudolf Steiner's anthroposophy and see measles merely as a harmless childhood disease and, simultaneously, as a necessary stage in the process of development from child to adulthood—on par with losing primary teeth. They might even be convinced that exposure to measles serves the best interest of their child. However, other parents insist on forgoing vaccination because they are seeking to carve out all-natural lives for their children, to maintain their purity, or to avoid contamination, assuming that vaccines contain toxic preservatives such as the mercury-based thimerosal.[4] What unites these parents is that they dispute the evidence of mainstream science that confirms vaccines are safe and effective; instead, they argue that immunization is much more dangerous than the risk of contracting the disease.[5] Their view of what is best for their child shares some of the core values of a "basic interests" standard—notably that a child's health is to be protected—but they disagree with the scientific basis of specific interventions that protect health.

In these discussions, vaccine-critical parents typically conflate two arguments. The first is that decisions about childhood vaccination should only be determined by the interests of the child involved; the second is that this implies that they, as parents, have the ultimate authority to determine what these interests are. However, these two claims are independent, and there is no reason why someone who accepts the first claim must also accept the second. We have already argued that vaccination serves a public good and therefore should not solely be evaluated from the perspective of the interests of the individual child. But even if we do view vaccination decisions in terms of an individual child's interest, that does not imply that it is always up to parents to decide. Of course, as we explained in section 3.8, respect for parental autonomy is important. Government should not interfere unnecessarily in the parent–child relationship. It is also firmly embedded in international conventions. Article 18 of the International Covenant on Civil and Political Rights (ICCPR) protects the right to freedom of thought, conscience, and religion, while article 18(4) states that "the States Parties to the present Covenant undertake to have respect for the liberty of parents . . . to ensure the religious and moral education of their children in conformity with their own convictions." Article 2 of the First Protocol to the European Convention on Human Rights states, "In the exercise of any functions which it assumes in relation to education and to teaching, the State shall respect the right of parents to ensure such education and teaching in conformity with their own religious and philosophical convictions."

At the same time, and as argued previously, article 3 of the UNCRC directs states to protect the basic interests of children who cannot yet make a well-informed decision on vaccination. A prudent government policy strikes a reasonable balance between two rights: on the one hand, there is the right of nonvaccinating parents to raise their children according to their deeply held convictions and the corresponding duty of the government not to interfere with these parental choices. On the other hand, there is the right of the child to have their basic interests protected and to grow up in good health, including being protected against avoidable diseases—with the corresponding duty of the government to protect the rights of the child. The question that emerges, then, is under which circumstances should the state's responsibility to protect a child's basic interests overrule the right of parents to follow their deeply felt desire not to vaccinate?

5.3   Parental Prerogative or *Parens Patriae*? The Harm Threshold

It is generally taken for granted in liberal-democratic regimes that parents have the primary prerogative in the upbringing of their children. Neutrality requires the state to be agnostic toward the myriad ideas about the good life that parents may endorse, including their ideas about what is best for their children. Moreover, it is in the interests of both parents and children that government does not unnecessarily interfere in the privacy of family life and the parent–child relationship as protected by, for example, article 8 of the ECHR.

Still, there remains a difference between the freedom of parents to live their own life in line with their idea of the good life and their freedom to raise their children as they like. Parents act as fiduciaries and guardians for their children, who are not yet capable of making deliberate choices—a role that slowly dissolves as the child approaches adulthood. Yet, from the very start at (or even before) birth, parenthood comes primarily with the obligation to protect the ongoing interests of children as vulnerable and maturing moral human beings who are in the process of developing into self-reliant persons.[6] Parental autonomy is not a self-standing right; it is a right that parents have *in their role* as parents and fiduciaries and in their endeavor of guiding their offspring toward independence. After all, children are neither an extension of their parents nor valid objects of their parents' self-expression. Instead, they are "self-originating sources of valid claims" (Rawls, 1980, p. 543). If parents fail to take on their role as parents responsibly, the state has a responsibility to intervene.

So, on the one hand, the state usually delegates its initial responsibility for children's basic interests to parents, working from the assumption that the decisions parents make follow their idea of what is best for their child and that this in turn also promotes the child's basic interests. Given the fact that most parents care deeply about their children and interact with them on a day-to-day basis, they will usually be better situated than any other actor, including the state, to understand the unique needs of their children and to make decisions that are in their children's best interests. On the other hand, the state never fully relinquishes final authority over a child's basic interests. Instead, it assumes a secondary and inverted role. It leaves most choices concerning child-rearing to parents and only interferes actively in parental autonomy when it is evident that a child's basic interests are (about to be) harmed because of parental decisions. That is, the state employs a "harm threshold," below which state interference is necessary and justified when basic interests are about to be harmed (Birchley, 2016a, 2016b; Diekema, 2004).

This concept of the "harm threshold" is, of course, a straightforward contextual application of Mill's harm principle that we introduced in chapter 4 as the main justification for liberty-limiting policies. The freedom of parents to raise their children in line with their ideas of the good life is limited, since it should not result in the avoidable risk of harm to their children, death, or lifelong disability, and the state has an obligation to intervene to protect the infant when this can be done easily and safely (cf. Dawson, 2011, p. 146). The doctrine of *parens patriae* allows state interference to protect a child's basic interests, iconically established as a legal principle by the US Supreme Court in *Prince v. Massachusetts* (1943): "Parents may be free to become martyrs themselves. But it does not follow that they are free, in identical circumstances, to make martyrs of their children."

In a recent case, the European Court argued that "the obligation on States to place the best interests of the child . . . at the center of all decisions affecting their health and development" concerns the interests of not only the child involved but all children as a group:

When it comes to immunisation, the objective should be that every child is protected against serious diseases. In the great majority of cases, this is achieved by children receiving the full schedule of vaccinations during their early years. Those to whom such treatment cannot be administered are indirectly protected against contagious diseases as long as the requisite level of vaccination coverage is maintained in their community, i.e. their protection comes from herd immunity. ("Vavřička," 2021, p. 65, ¶288)

In pluralistic liberal democracies, the state can only have legitimate authority to ensure the basic interests of children if empirical claims about what does or does not contribute to health and well-being are truly independent and devoid of commitments to specific worldviews. Moreover, given that this authority may imply overruling parents' choices, judgments about the basic interests of children should be based on the best possible biomedical evidence. Hence, as far as the contribution of vaccination to a child's health is concerned, democratic governments will make decisions by appealing to the state of scientific knowledge about vaccination and not to anthroposophist or other worldviews. Given that there is a broad scientific consensus that diseases like measles, polio, and pertussis can have very serious—lethal or permanently disabling—complications and that vaccinations against these infections are effective and safe, it is reasonable to hold that such vaccinations do indeed protect a basic interest of each child.

This argument provides an answer to the question posed in the last section: under which circumstances is the protection of the child's basic interests a ground for the government to override the rights of parents to follow their (deeply felt) desire not to vaccinate? Even though parental prerogative is the most plausible starting point for this discussion, it is never an absolute principle. The doctrine of *parens patriae* holds that the state has its own responsibility to ensure that the basic interests of all children are secured. Its application in a specific case may be debatable, but the concept of *parens patriae* itself is not suspect in the least (Reiss, 2015, p. 3). At the end of the day, the state has a responsibility to safeguard each child's basic interests, including the interest of being free from preventable diseases. The child's basic interests define a *harm threshold* that sets limits on the freedom of parents to raise their children according to their conception of the good life. The harm threshold thus functions as an emergency brake on the parental prerogative, and this is especially the case if there is an avoidable risk of serious long-term or permanent injury or death (Dawson, 2005, p. 78).

This conclusion is in line with—*and endorses*—a central principle of modern constitutional thought, which is that the state must have the ultimate *Kompetenz-Kompetenz*. This is the competence to rule as to the extent of its own competence on when this is contested and, thus, to determine the respective areas of competence of natural persons and associations within its jurisdiction (Laborde, 2017, pp. 160–196). The state has the competence to determine the respective areas of competence of natural persons and associations within its jurisdiction. It is the state that provides parents with the legal right to the freedom of thought, conscience, and religion and the subsequent parental prerogative to raise their children in line with their ideas of what is good for their child. However, it is also the state that determines *the limits* of these fundamental rights and freedoms, especially when they clash with other fundamental rights and freedoms—including the rights of children to have their basic interests protected. Only governmental agencies can unilaterally determine the range and limits of the rights and duties of (associations of) citizens within their jurisdiction (Laborde, 2017, pp. 160–196). In summary, the state has the ultimate competence to employ the harm threshold as an emergency brake on parental prerogative when the basic interests of children are (about to be) harmed. The next question, regarding in which circumstances the government should be pulling this emergency brake, will be answered in subsequent sections.

5.4 The Harm Threshold and Refusal of Blood Transfusion

Let us take stock: parents have the primary prerogative in the upbringing of their children and in ensuring that their children's basic interests and best interests are taken care of. At the same time, the state never fully relinquishes final authority over a child's basic interests. It employs a harm threshold, leaving most choices concerning child-rearing to parents, and only intervenes if it is clear that a child's basic interests are about to be harmed. Let's explore a well-known problem in clinical ethics to elucidate how this harm threshold works in real-life cases, before getting back to vaccination. A commonly discussed case, both in medical ethics and law, is about Jehovah's Witnesses refusing blood transfusion. Jehovah's Witnesses see blood transfusions as a violation of certain passages in the Bible (e.g., Acts 15:20 and 15:28–29) that call for "abstaining from blood." In modern medicine, an adult person's decision to reject a (medically necessary) blood transfusion will often be respected. As argued in section 3.6, the right to bodily integrity makes it almost impossible to override a competent person's choice to refuse medical treatment. However, if it is about blood transfusion for a young child (e.g., a newborn with rhesus disease), the story will be different. Rhesus disease (also known as hemolytic disease) is a condition where antibodies in a pregnant woman's blood destroy her baby's blood cells. In severe cases, a newborn baby will need a blood transfusion to survive. Courts in liberal democracies recognize parental autonomy in medical decisions but "additionally recognize that these rights are not absolute and exist only to promote the welfare of children." (Wolley, 2005, p. 715). In situations where doctors or other care providers consider the medical treatment necessary because of a clear and present danger of severe harm, they cannot simply accept a refusal of permission by parents. Western legal systems address parental refusal of blood transfusions by requiring doctors to notify the judicial authorities. These authorities may override parents' wishes about treatment of their child or even temporarily remove their parental rights (Conti et al., 2018, p. 102) to ensure that the child will be given blood.

This provides a good explanation of how the harm threshold works. In normal health care contexts, physicians will not treat children without their parents' permission, and they will support parents to come to a decision that is in the best interests of their child. Health care providers and parents will often jointly decide what is best. Ultimately, parents have wide discretion to observe their child's best interests and make (medical) decisions for their child, and if there is not a complete consensus between doctors and parents about which of several treatment options is preferred, physicians will normally defer to the parents' judgment. Yet parents do not have an absolute right to refuse medical treatment, and if physicians are convinced that refusal will be harmful for the child, for example, because there is a risk of death or permanent disability, they should diverge from the parents' view of the best interests of the child. The fact that parents have religious reasons for their refusal does not make a difference in such a case (Wolley, 2005, p. 716). Physicians can start a legal procedure and ask the judge for permission to administer medical treatment. The case of a Jehovah's Witness rhesus baby is relatively straightforward because blood transfusion is a curative medical intervention that is a necessary life-saving response to an imminent lethal risk. If the harm threshold is surpassed, the state has the ultimate authority to determine the limits of parental authority and the statutory legitimacy to override parental choices. But, as just argued, this is an emergency-break procedure, which is applied only in exceptional situations. One can think of many medical procedures that, although important for a child's current and future health, do not surpass this harm threshold. Especially in the case of preventive care, it is not obvious that the risks to be prevented are great enough to warrant restricting parental autonomy. This is not to say that such prevention is unimportant, but if enforcing prevention involves overriding parental choice, this is only clearly justified when there is an imminent threat of severe harm.

5.5   Is Vaccination a Basic Interest?

The state has a responsibility to observe basic rights of children, and in extreme cases, this may imply that choices of parents are overruled. Blood transfusion for Jehovah's Witness babies with rhesus disease is a clear case. But can immunization be considered analogously? Are vaccinations to be considered as protecting a basic interest of children, and if so, does that imply that public health authorities (possibly via a court order) are justified in setting aside the concerns of parents who would refuse immunization for their child?

Most immunizations, like many other forms of medical treatment, are indeed concerned with a *basic* interest, that is, being protected against serious (potentially lethal or disabling) diseases. Of course, parents may have different views of the seriousness of those diseases or the safety of the procedure; even if they acknowledge that adverse effects are rare, they may fear that their child will be unlucky in this respect. People who endorse an anthroposophist view of life often see "childhood diseases" like measles or pertussis as a meaningful step in child development, and vaccinations in their view do not optimally contribute to a child's well-being. This shows how empirical claims about what does or does not contribute to health can be embedded in metaphysical assumptions or specific conceptions of what the good life consists of. Such assumptions are inevitable in any comprehensive idea of what determines a person's (i.e., a child's) best interest. However, we are not concerned with judgments about *what is best for children* that allow for strong commitments to a specific idea of the good life but with *basic interests* that apply to any person—regardless of their (parents') religion or conception of the good life. In a democratic, pluralistic state, the government can only have legitimate authority to ensure the basic interests of children if it can ground claims about the safety and effectiveness of interventions on sound and uncontroversial scientific evidence and state-of-the-art medical practice. Given that there is a very broad scientific consensus that diseases like measles, polio, and pertussis can have very serious—lethal or permanently disabling—complications and that vaccinations against these infections are effective and safe, it is reasonable to hold that such vaccinations do indeed protect a basic interest of each child.

Yet this claim—that common childhood immunizations protect a child's *basic* interest—does not necessarily imply that immunizations can also be enforced against the will of parents. Exploring the analogy with the Jehovah's Witness blood transfusion case is, again, instructive. What makes that case exceptional is that it involves a *necessary* response to an *imminent, life-threatening* risk. Childhood immunization programs do protect against disease that can be life threatening or disabling, but compared to the blood transfusion case, the risk is, at least in normal times, much, much smaller. Immunization offers protection if the person being vaccinated will be exposed to a pathogen like measles, but thanks to successful collective immunization programs, many people may never be exposed to that pathogen.

There are cases in which immunization offers the only genuinely effective protection against an imminent and serious threat—namely, when an unvaccinated child has been exposed to a potentially lethal or disabling pathogen such as measles or hepatitis B. In such a case, prophylactic immunization given within a couple of days may prevent infection or prevent the most severe symptoms. There are different forms of postexposure prophylaxis (passive immunization by administering immunoglobin or active immunization by administering a regular vaccine), but both can be considered effective responses to an imminent, serious threat to a child's life and health. Prophylactic immunization after exposure to a pathogen thus has some of the central features of the Jehovah's Witness blood transfusion case, which supports seeing it as protecting a child's basic interest, and thus also as an intervention that public health authorities could enforce against the will of parents. Arguably, the health of a rhesus baby in need of blood transfusion is still much more severely threatened than the health of an unvaccinated child who is exposed to measles. Nevertheless, unprotected exposure to a lethal pathogen is thwarting a basic interest, and this implies that the state should interfere immediately if effective protection is available.[7]

Note that in such a case, *forced vaccination* would be necessary, which is the most intrusive measure in our categorization of interventions (section 2.4), involving the clearest and strictest limitation of parental autonomy. It completely bypasses parental discretion: parental autonomy is not merely constrained; it is eliminated. Most discussions about setting limits on parental freedom to refuse vaccination are not, however, about forced vaccination but about policies that set vaccination as a requirement for school entry, or for child benefits, or that make vaccination refusal a criminal offense. Such policies, even though they are mandatory or compulsory, still leave opportunities for parents to be exempted or to otherwise avoid vaccination of their child. For that reason, these less intrusive alternatives will be irrelevant for a government that has a *pro tanto* obligation *to secure* protection and thus enforce vaccination as a basic interest for a child at immediate risk.

Our conclusion is that childhood immunization does protect the basic interests of children that the state must guarantee, but that, in normal times, the risks of nonvaccination are too remote to warrant forced vaccination against the will of parents. The analogy with the blood transfusion case does not make sense in the case of routine immunization programs. It only makes sense in cases of *postexposure prophylactic* immunization or during an outbreak of a lethal disease where exposure cannot be avoided. Outside the context of an immediate and possibly lethal threat of infection, there is no place for forced vaccinations. This is not only because in normal circumstances, the risk for each individual child will be remote, but also because there is an alternative way for the government to protect each child's basic interests in normal conditions: by maintaining adequate collective protection via high vaccination rates.

Our analysis in terms of basic and best interests of children thus offers additional support for policies that aim at group-level protection. Maintaining such group protection is necessary for the state to fulfill a key responsibility: to secure basic interests of all children. In circumstances of robust herd immunity, parents do not expose their own child to an unacceptable risk if they refuse vaccination, and then *forced* immunization would be unwarranted. However, they do undermine the collective endeavor to maintain the group-level protection that is benefiting their child as well. Hence, as argued already in the previous chapter, vaccination refusal does fall within the scope of the harm principle, and this offers support for mandatory or compulsory programs.

5.6   Basic and Best Interests in Childhood Immunization: A Conclusion

In this chapter, we have argued that in most cases, most of the time, it is parents and not the state who have the authority to determine what is in the best interests of their young children, and they have the freedom and responsibility to act in line with their view of what is best for their child. Parents' views on this matter can, however, conflict with their child's *basic* interests, and the protection of basic interests is ultimately a responsibility for the state. Basic interests are those interests that are deemed necessary for a very broad range of opportunities in current and later life—and hence are consistent with and necessary for a broad variety of conceptions of the good life. They include interests such as being protected from serious diseases, being adequately nourished, growing up in a safe environment in which caring relations can flourish, and having access to a good-quality education.

Threats to a child's basic interests are always a sufficient reason for the state to intervene, to protect the child or enable parents to do so. But if a basic interest of a child is at stake due to the choices or actions of the parents themselves, the state will be reluctant to intervene in family life and overrule parental decisions. This is because parental autonomy and freedom of religion or belief are core values in a democratic society. Overruling these values requires a thorough weighing up of all competing interests, taking all contextual factors into account, such as the magnitude of the risk, the nature of the intervention, and the availability of alternative measures to protect the child.

In the case of Jehovah's Witnesses who refuse medically necessary blood transfusions for their newborn child, legal intervention is justified (temporarily) to remove the child from the custody of parents so that they can receive the treatment they need. The treatment is necessary to avert a present danger in the form of a life-threatening disease, so this is a relatively clear case. Vaccination is more complex because it is a preventive intervention that takes away a risk that is often remote. Nevertheless, we claim that the analogy with parents refusing blood transfusion can largely be upheld if parents refuse vaccination of their child who is at *immediate* risk of infection with a *serious* (life-threatening or disabling) disease. Even though the risk will be still much smaller in the extreme vaccination case compared to the blood transfusion case, we hold that it passes the harm threshold and thus warrants government force.

Hence, we conclude that there are cases, probably only during an outbreak, where the state is ethically justified in overruling parental refusal and enforcing immunization of a young child. This can best be done by a court ruling relating to individual children rather than a sweeping policy drafted by public health care authorities, ensuring that there are relevant checks and balances and a fair procedure. Outside the context of an outbreak, forced vaccination against infectious diseases is difficult to justify—not only because the risk of infection as such will be much smaller but also because health authorities will have other, more proportionate measures that they can implement to protect the basic interests of all children: a mandatory or compulsory vaccination program that is sufficiently coercive—but not more than necessary—to maintain high immunization rates.

6 Mandatory Childhood Vaccination and Legal Exemptions

In chapter 4, we offered a principled argument claiming that governments are justified in imposing liberty-limiting vaccination policies when this is necessary to prevent harm to others. We introduced Mill's harm principle, which offers a basic justification for justifying liberty-limiting vaccination policies, even if this involves a restriction of such basic rights as freedom of conscience, thought, or religion and the right to family life. In chapter 5, we explained what this implies for vaccination programs for young children. We translated the more general "harm principle" into the "harm threshold" and concluded that under specific circumstances, government is allowed (and required) to interfere in parental prerogative.

However, the question remains in which situations such infringement of the fundamental rights of parents is necessary and proportionate. If herd protection can still be established or maintained in ways that leave parental freedoms intact, this will certainly be preferable. In this chapter, we explore a first possible way for states to opt for a proportionate policy—namely, by making childhood vaccination compulsory (enforced by punitive sanctions) or mandatory (by, for example, requiring it for school entry) while tolerating a small group of refusers by allowing them to apply for *nonmedical exemptions*.

The maintenance of herd protection, like that of many other public goods, does not require that every person in the target group complies. To prevent or contain outbreaks and stop the transmission of a highly contagious pathogen, it will be sufficient to have an approximately 95 percent immunization coverage. This figure applies to measles, which is one of the diseases that spreads most easily within a naive population. Other pathogens are less infectious, and for these, herd protection is possible at a somewhat lower vaccination rate, such as 80–86 percent for diphtheria (RIVM, 2019).

If robust herd protection is established, everyone enjoys protection, including vulnerable persons who are not (yet) vaccinated or for other reasons are susceptible to infection. If incomplete coverage, say 95 percent, is sufficient, this leaves room to accommodate noncompliance and tolerate people who have deeply held convictions that require them to refuse vaccination. This can be done by allowing them to be exempted from the otherwise compulsory program. Is this a viable and justifiable policy option for constitutional liberal-democratic regimes?

6.1 Rule-and-Exemption Policies

Over time, liberal political orders have endorsed and implemented *rule-and-exemption* policies as a way of dealing with legal obligations regarding morally sensitive issues. This is a legal arrangement that imposes a uniform rule on all citizens to do specific things, while simultaneously granting exemptions to designated minorities who can show that complying with the rule would severely burden them by requiring them to act against their conscience or prevent them from engaging in important symbolic practices (Miller, 2014, p. 438). A well-known example is the exemption from compulsory military service for conscientious objectors. Childhood vaccination is a similarly sensitive issue. Even though a large majority of parents participate voluntarily— and often wholeheartedly—in childhood vaccination programs, a minority has strong objections to such programs. Could there be a way to maintain collective protection through herd immunity and simultaneously accommodate the interests of those who deeply object to vaccination?

Historically, these legal exemptions originated in Western liberal democracies as religious exemptions available only to a very limited category of members of recognized religions. In 1928, the Dutch government created the option for parents to be exempted from smallpox immunization, which at that time was compulsory and backed up by financial penalties. The exemption could be granted by the mayor of their municipality, who was expected to consider the trustworthiness of parents' religious grounds for objection. Over time, the policy shifted from compulsory to mandatory, and the exemption became available to a wider category of parents. In many countries, however, governments still distinguish religious from secular (or "philosophical") objections.

Maybe the best-known existing examples of immunization *rule-and-exemption* policies are those allowing waivers in the United States. There is no federal regulation, but all US states legally require the vaccination of children prior to school or day care entry.[1] These mandatory policies began at the end of the nineteenth century, when some US states started to require schoolchildren to be vaccinated against smallpox. By the late 1960s, many states also required schoolchildren to be vaccinated against measles. Over the following decades, states added to the list of vaccines that were mandated for children enrolling in school (and, later, day care) (Navin, 2018, p. 186). This requirement was accompanied by a system of medical, religious, and philosophical exemptions. The US federal exemption jurisprudence allows states to give vaccination waivers but does not mandate it (Reiss, 2014, p. 1563).

Around 2015, these exemptions became subject to scrutiny in California as it became clear that the Disneyland measles outbreak was caused by substandard vaccination compliance due to high numbers of nonmedical exemptions. In reaction to the outbreak and the public outrage it generated, the state of California passed a bill that eliminated all nonmedical exemptions. Legislators in some other states also introduced bills that would make it harder for parents to opt out of vaccinating their kids. As a result, these exemptions, which were virtually undisputed for a long time, have now become the subject of intense public and political discussion.

6.2 Three Requirements for Rule-and-Exemption Policies

How should the accommodation of exemptions be judged in the context of constitutional liberal democracies? At first sight, allowing exemptions seems to contradict a basic requirement of the idea of constitutional democracy. After all, clear application of the law, equal treatment, and the rule of law are paramount; law ought to be administered impartially and should have no favorites (Barry, 2001; Trigg, 2012). At the same time, the liberal state should acknowledge that apparently neutral laws might nevertheless be disproportionally more burdensome for certain citizens than for others. Even though most parents comply voluntarily with the duty to vaccinate, some parents have deep objections to the practice. Nonvoluntary vaccination implies that these parents must go against their conscience or have to sacrifice deep commitments. And even though most other citizens do not share these convictions—or might even object to them—they might nevertheless understand the importance of the convictions for the individual person that holds them and acknowledge the pain it will inflict on parents if they have to act against their deepest commitments about what is best for their child.

The question, then, is when universal application of law must be paramount and under which circumstances exemptions should prevail. This has been a central question in the political-theoretical debates of the past two decades on legal exemptions. So-called muscular liberals rally around the idea of universal egalitarian law and argue that law, as the outcome of democratic deliberation and political processes, should, in principle, be administered impartially and be universally binding. Brian Barry's *Culture and Equality* (2001) is arguably the best-known placeholder for this position. Other liberal authors, however, see legal exemptions to universal laws as the contemporary interpretation of the ancient liberal ideal of toleration (Dobbernack & Modood, 2013; Forst, 2012; Williams, 1996). They would argue that a blanket application of state law sometimes unduly burdens citizens who deeply disagree with the law because it fundamentally contradicts their conscience and deepest convictions. Allowing exemptions recognizes this fact by alleviating the particular burden of the members of these minority groups.

We do not aim to take a firm theoretical position in this more political-theoretical debate.[2] We assume that the idea of accommodation fits, *ipso facto*, with the central tenets of constitutional liberal democracy, especially in cases in which granting exemptions does not directly violate the fundamental rights and basic interests of others.[3] The fact that herd immunity can be maintained at a vaccination rate of approximately 95 percent implies that there might be quite some room for exemptions from compulsory vaccination without endangering public health and the rights of others. We agree with Mahoney (2011, p. 311) that government should seek to accommodate minority practices in the most generous manner possible. It should be clear, though, what kind of entitlement the granting of vaccine exemptions involves. It is not a straightforward and inviolable right of parents that nullifies the duty to vaccinate; instead, it is a toleration-based and conditional right to an *exemption* from a general legal duty, which can and should be revoked when robust herd immunity is endangered (Nehushtan, 2012). Thus, in the rest of the chapter, we take for granted that *rule-and-exemption* policies are not necessarily required by central liberal-democratic values but, in principle, also do not contradict liberal-democratic values. However, when they are implemented, they should not undermine the very same principles.

Indeed, to be feasible, rule-and-exemption policies need to comply with three requirements simultaneously: the limitation requirement, the justice requirement, and the distinctiveness requirement. Let us discuss these three requirements in turn. The *limitation requirement* determines that the number of exemptions allowed is limited; these should not be so numerous that they undermine or nullify the goal for which the specific legal duty has been introduced. Exemptions to legal duties can only be maintained if a large majority of citizens have sufficient reason to endorse and abide by the law (Vallier, 2016) and only a small minority seeks an exemption. Second, the *justice requirement* acknowledges that exemptions are scarce goods that are given to some and withheld from others. This distribution of exemptions should not be unjust, for example, by privileging or discriminating against certain religious or nonreligious doctrines or by unduly undermining the ideal of state neutrality.[4] Third, a policy needs to satisfy the *distinctiveness requirement*, which implies that exemptions can only be granted if it is possible for government agencies, in the judicial fact-finding process, to distinguish between sincere and deeply held objections against the requirement that is imposed on people and mere "exemptions of convenience." Moreover, to be transparent and to avoid making arbitrary decisions, government agencies should be able to make such distinctions by applying relatively straightforward legal rules.

When applied to immunization policies, the limitation requirement implies that coverage should be sufficient to ensure a group-level protection that is necessary to prevent outbreaks and protect vulnerable persons. Moreover, the average vaccination rate should not only be high enough to protect vulnerable individuals within the population as a whole, but coverage should also be such that local pockets of undervaccination are small enough to minimize the risk of outbreaks within such pockets. Whereas the limitation requirement is linked to the core objectives of the policy, the other two are general requirements for fair policies. If vaccine exemptions are granted, the separation of sincere objections and less-sincere objections should not violate central liberal values, for example, by discriminating against specific religious doctrines, and the process of granting exemptions must be based on verifiable legal rules. Only if all three requirements are met is a mandatory vaccination scheme with waivers, all things considered, justifiable.

In the next section, we argue that this leads to a paradox for liberal-democratic exemption policies for mandatory childhood vaccination law, because it appears to be impossible to satisfy all three requirements simultaneously. The policy of accepting categories of objectors is neutral, which would open the door to too many exemption claims that would in turn endanger robust herd immunity. Or the number of categories of objectors must be limited, which cannot be done in a neutral and feasible way, thus violating the other two requirements. This leads to the conclusion that it is *impossible* to maintain a system of vaccine waivers for the measles vaccination that is both consistent with central liberal-democratic tenets and also leaves robust herd immunity intact.

6.3   The Impossibility of Satisfying All Requirements

The limitation requirement sets limits on the number of exemptions that can be granted. In our assessment of a threshold vaccination rate, we should take into consideration that part of the "space" is already taken up by persons who cannot (yet) undergo vaccination for medical reasons: infants who have not yet completed the recommended childhood immunization schedule and persons who cannot undergo vaccination for medical reasons because they have certain forms of cancer, have a compromised immune system, or are likely to have a serious allergic reaction. These exemptions are medical necessities and should be given priority over nonmedical exemptions: persons who have a medical condition that does not allow them to be vaccinated cannot reasonably be required to do so, but everyone else can be. Protecting the health of the former should be given priority above allowing the latter an exemption to what they are normally required to do anyway. The number of medical exemptions will be low, however: a recent study in Arkansas found only 0.01 percent of medical vaccine exemptions among students from preschool to college (Safi et al., 2012). This suggests that there is still ample room for allowing nonmedical exemptions.

However, we should also take into account that vaccination rates are not distributed evenly across a nation; each state or region may contain local pockets of undervaccination. Moreover, these requests for exemptions will also not be distributed evenly across a society but will be concentrated precisely within these pockets of undervaccination. There is therefore an increased risk of local breakdowns of herd protection and disease outbreaks within these "hotspots" (May & Silverman, 2003; Yang & Debold, 2014).[5]

In theory, this could imply that, somewhat counterintuitively, fewer exemptions can be granted in areas in which the number of people who object to immunization for religious or other reasons is relatively high. On the other hand, it is obvious that at the same time, the more groups opposing vaccination have their exemption claims legally accepted, the more unlikely it becomes that the limitation requirement is fulfilled. A historical analysis of US jurisprudence regarding the waiver system can illuminate that.[6] Historically, the number of exemptions granted was limited because only a very specific category of objectors was eligible: members of nationally recognized and established religious denominations. In 1971, several state courts widened the domain of exemptions "to everyone and anyone who claims a sincerely held religious belief."[7] Only in 1979 was the privileged position of religion disputed in court, because religious exemptions "discriminate against the great majority of children whose parents have no such religious convictions."[8]

It makes sense to remove the distinction between religious and secular claims for exemptions, because it does not fit with current, more secular ideals that suggest governments should be neutral toward various (religious and secular) ideas of the good life (Pierik & Van der Burg, 2014). Moreover, the original distinction led to many odd exceptions. For example, although many secular claims were not even taken into consideration, an exemption claimed by a Jewish parent was allowed by a US court, even though nothing in Judaism supports objections to vaccinations (Calandrillo, 2004, p. 414, n 388). Another example is the fact that thousands of parents have qualified for religious exemptions by joining sham mail-order religions such as the Congregation of Universal Wisdom, through a contribution of $75 and a $15 fee for the official notification necessary to qualify for the exemption. The main article of faith of the Congregation, quite characteristically, is that the injection of any medication or other humanmade substance would violate the sanctity of the body (McNeil, 2003).

From the perspective of the justice requirement, this historical development of an ever-more inclusive approach can only be encouraged. The growing focus on state neutrality and secular law in the past few decades affects the way such claims to exemptions are assessed. The more secular the assessment of exemption claims becomes, the more difficult and problematic it is to distinguish religious from nonreligious convictions and, more important, to distinguish "strong beliefs" from "mere preferences." In the liberal tradition, one that is determined so much by inter-Christian strife in Europe after the Reformation, such strong beliefs and the mere concepts of "conscience" and "conscientious objections" were limited to the quite contingent category of members of nationally recognized and established Christian denominations and very much understood in terms of Christian terminology and symbolism (Spinner-Halev, 2005; Waldron, 1987). In current, more secular times, we need a more inclusive conception of the "strong beliefs" and "deep commitments" that provides a normative status to convictions that individuals closely identify with and recognize as theirs, on the grounds of their "deep," "serious," and "spiritual" nature. After all, it is because these religious and secular commitments meet the criterion of deep commitments that they justify exemptions from universal law.[9]

This more inclusive approach can be recognized in current jurisprudence of the US Supreme Court and the European Court of Human Rights. In *US v. Seeger*, the US Supreme Court abandoned, for matters concerning conscientious objection to military service, the religious/secular distinction by holding that an objection can be understood as "religious" when it is based on a "sincere and meaningful belief which occupies in the life of its possessor a place parallel to that filled by the God of those."[10] Following this jurisprudence, it is remarkable that several US states still only accept religious exemptions and deny secular exemptions; one would expect the distinction to have collapsed as soon as a secular parent in one of these states made a case before the Supreme Court. However, it turns out that *Seeger* was an exception because the Supreme Court was interpreting the narrow terms of a statute rather than addressing the constitutional question of what should count as protected belief for purposes of the Free Exercise Clause of the First Amendment. As a result, judges have been reluctant to extend the constitutional protection of nonreligious deep, serious, moral commitments beyond narrowly circumscribed cases of conscientious objection to military service (Laborde, 2014, p. 68). Mark Navin concludes that the separation between religious and non-religious claims has lost much of its relevance in US jurisprudence because more systematic nonreligious commitments are also considered religious—whether they are based in a theistic belief or moral conscience. The only condition is that they must play "an important role in a person's ability to realize personal integrity" (Navin, 2018, p. 196). For many who reject vaccination, this is only one element of a larger set of practices that also includes extended breastfeeding, organic cooking, and homeschooling. Therefore, this way of parenting is best described as a comprehensive life project that plays an important role in a person's idea of integrity. In a similar way, Micah Schwartzman (2012, p. 1421) argues that we have good reason to endorse a "definitional expansion" of religion to also include nontheistic commitments. If the US Constitution prioritizes exemptions for religious objectors, this expansion might be needed to achieve state neutrality toward theistic and nontheistic commitments.

The European Court of Human Rights, which was established only in 1959, never provided a comprehensive definition of the term "religion" or "belief." Mainstream religions were always accepted as belief systems; the court merely employs formal criteria to other religions and personal belief systems: the conviction must display "a certain level of cogency, seriousness, cohesion, and importance."[11] These terms have never been spelled out in case law, but Murdoch (2007, p. 11) explains that a specific act, that is, objecting to vaccination, must relate to a weighty and substantial aspect of human life and behavior and be deemed worthy of protection in European democratic society.[12] But nothing in these formulations separates religious from secular convictions.

For liberal governments to comply with the contemporary demands of state neutrality—and for the US government to comply with the Free Exercise Clause of the First Amendment—the earlier theistic and substantial interpretation of the term "religious" must be abandoned and replaced by a more inclusive and formal one. This is also clear when we analyze the myriad of claims to exemptions from childhood vaccination today. Should modern objectors who, in one spiritual way or another, still adhere to Wakefield's debunked claim that vaccination causes autism as discussed in section 3.3, be treated differently from Christians who argue that vaccination is an inappropriate meddling in the work of God, or from those who argue that diseases should be healed through prayer instead of medication, or from metaphysical thinkers who argue that vaccines undermine "purity" or hamper "spiritual growth of the person"? Yes, the commitment of the "modern objector" is based on a factual claim that contradicts evidence-based medicine, while the more clearly religious objections cannot be refuted scientifically at all, but this is as such not sufficient as a criterion that can be employed by a neutral state for distinguishing the two types of claims or to conclude that one justifies an exemption while the other does not. Moreover, modern antivaccination beliefs are usually embedded in a broader worldview that includes normative and metaphysical beliefs about what is natural and how living according to nature is conducive to health, as well as strong opinions about health risks and the trustworthiness of mainstream science and "Big Pharma." This further undermines a clear-cut distinction between comprehensive views of life, such as a religion, and personal judgments about the necessity and safety of vaccines.

This is all very much in line with the justice requirement described earlier. Exemptions are scarce goods, and their distribution should not privilege or discriminate against certain religious or nonreligious doctrines or unduly undermine the ideal of state neutrality.

The discussion so far also shows that there are severe tensions between the three requirements just discussed. First, the justice requirement and the limitation requirement cannot be held simultaneously. The justice requirement demands an inclusive and formal approach to religious and nonreligious ideas of the good life. However, as more categories of exemption claimers are accepted, more persons can claim exemptions and the more the limitation requirement is endangered. It appears that the requirements cannot all be satisfied simultaneously. This leads to a paradox: the pre-1971 substantial formulation limiting exemptions to members of nationally recognized and established religious denominations might comply with the limitation requirement but falls short on the justice requirement; conversely, the approach focusing on the level of cogency, seriousness, cohesion, and importance does comply with the justice requirement but might not satisfy the limitation requirement.

Moreover, there are good reasons to assume that the justice requirement no longer fits well with the distinctiveness requirement, which demands that government agencies should be able to *distinguish* between sincere objections against vaccination and so-called exemptions of convenience. The more formal—rather than substantive—the criteria become, the more the distinction between religious and philosophical convictions evaporates. That is in line with the justice requirement, but it has an unintended effect. Once the distinction between religious and secular objections cannot be made meaningfully, separating sincere objections and mere exemptions of convenience is also "beyond the practical and institutional competence of courts" (Dane, 1980, p. 350). If law, policy, and adjudication can no longer rely on substantial criteria and have to fall back on formal criteria like sincerity, cogency, or cohesion, it will become impossible for government agencies to separate genuine claims from those of consistent free riders, and this means that the distinctiveness requirement is not met.

Moreover, if only formal criteria are employed, the waiver system will comply with the justice requirement, but it will also have to accept much more exemption claims. It will therefore be difficult to meet the limitation requirement: that a waiver system must be capable of limiting the number of exemptions to such an extent that herd immunity is not jeopardized. Again, when that distinction falls apart, it is also much harder to separate sincere objections from free rider claims disguised as sincere objections. This, in turn, makes it even more difficult to meet the limitation requirement. The more categories of exemption claimers that are acknowledged, the larger the number of (potential) claimants. If a liberal government aims to maintain herd immunity and if there is no neutral way of distinguishing insurmountable objections to vaccination from more superficial preferences, it will become very difficult to design a waiver system that is neutral toward different religious and secular ideas about the good life and is capable of maintaining robust herd immunity.

6.4 Procedural Approaches

In the previous sections, we concluded that it is very hard to substantively identify genuine objections to vaccination and, consequently, to design law and policies to distinguish genuine objections from exemptions of convenience. One way to hold on to a waiver system is to give up the attempt to substantively assess parental convictions and, instead, to employ a reasonable procedure to determine who can legitimately claim exemptions. The alternative service for conscientious objectors to the military service can serve as an example here. Recognized objectors must contribute to the public good in another way, for example, by serving in educational or health care institutions. In addition, the alternative service usually takes a longer period than the military service, up to twice as long, to deter insincere objectors from taking the alternative route. In our case of exemptions from vaccination, a similar path can be taken. Vaccinating one's children contributes to a public good and is burdensome to the parents and the child, although, as we argued in the previous chapter, for individuals, the burdens of vaccination are minor compared to the benefits. Alternative trajectories for vaccine objectors should contribute in a different way to the public good and/or should, in one way or another, be at least as onerous for parents as going through the vaccination procedure, to eliminate the easy way out of vaccination. The question is to what extent such an approach can comply with the requirements just formulated.

Let us discuss three procedural approaches. The first option is to require parents to follow a certain procedure before they are eligible for a vaccine waiver: to complete a set of educational sessions and to present their substantive opposition to vaccination before a formal review board. In this approach, the content of the objection is not substantially assessed; it is only marginally evaluated on whether it satisfies some basic formal requirements to qualify for an exemption from mandatory vaccination. The basic idea is that even though there is no substantive assessment of parents' arguments, the procedure forces them to become informed about the dangers of non-vaccination and to formulate their objections against vaccination explicitly and defend them in a formal setting. Even though undergoing this procedure might not substantially alter parents' beliefs about vaccination, at least it would make it harder for them to forgo vaccination without being confronted with information on the possible dangers involved. Mark Navin argues that it could be helpful to "redirect our attention away from the reasons people have for objecting, and focusing instead on the burdens they are willing to withstand in order to receive waivers" (Navin, 2016, p. 198). He argues that such measures may be burdensome enough to deter some parents from completing an application for a vaccine waiver. Moreover, he assumes that the "people who are most likely to be discouraged by more burdensome waiver application processes are likely to be people who have the least claim to receive exemptions in the first place" (Navin, 2016, p. 198).

The second procedure moves away from the problematic distinction between sincere objections and mere preferences by requiring that everyone should, in one way or another, contribute to the public good of herd immunity. The most obvious contribution is to vaccinate one's children (and oneself). Those with objections to vaccinations must contribute in another way, for example, through paying a tax that could finance vaccination schemes and thereby support vaccinations for low-income families. One advantage of this is that such a tax would be much less intrusive and might therefore be more acceptable for those with religious or philosophical objections. A second advantage is that such an approach would avoid the problem of assessing the true nature and depth of the objections. Your willingness to pay is taken as a proxy for the depth of your objections, and given the difficulty of determining sincere conscientious objections, willingness to pay might be the most neutral alternative. The level of taxation should yield a burden that is at least comparable with participating in a vaccination schedule to make sure that opting out is not less burdensome than participating. Perhaps the charge could be based on the expected damage, according to the *polluter pays principle*. Another calculation method would link the tax rate to the extent to which herd immunity is ensured in a certain area. If the number of objectors within a specific community is small, the tax rate can be low, only covering the administrative fee required to uphold the system of exemptions and monitor levels of herd immunity and possible outbreaks of infectious diseases. However, the larger the number of objectors in a specific area, the more the tax rate will rise. Willingness to pay could, in a way, be the most neutral way to separate the wheat from the chaff.

Lotteries might provide a third procedural approach. Peter Stone (2011) argues that lotteries are appropriately employed when it is essential to prevent irrelevant considerations affecting decisions about allocation of a certain good. If we conclude from the discussion so far that it is impossible to distinguish sincere objections from superficial preferences by relatively straightforward legal norms, we could distribute exemptions among parents who seek them through a lottery.

These procedures have several advantages. If they work, we can hold on to an exemption policy to ascertain that the mandatory vaccination scheme is proportionate. A second advantage is that government is discharged from the impossible task of substantively assessing the content or the depth of an objection to vaccination. At the same time, any policy that avoids a substantive assessment will probably be imperfect: it will allow too much if waivers are granted to parents who are only moderately opposed to vaccination, or it might exclude too much if waivers are denied to parents with genuine objections to vaccination who were unable to successfully pass the procedure (Navin, 2018, p. 201).

The first approach might not provide enough of a barrier to exemption claims to secure robust herd immunity. After all, if parents know they have to meet formal requirements but are in the end not assessed substantially, they know they just have to go through the motions to succeed. In addition, this approach will be biased in favor of educated people, who will find it easier to formulate their substantive opposition than less-educated people.

The second procedure might have the ability to limit the number of exemptions by raising the tax to the threshold level, but it has the disadvantage of being biased in favor of wealthier people, which arguably violates the justice requirement. In an unequal society, the tax will not distinguish sincere objections from reasons of convenience. Instead, it will just identify who is able to pay. If the tax is low, then we have done nothing to block the worries about exemptions of convenience for the better-off. If the tax is high, then only the better-off will be able to apply for exemptions. To the extent that we consider current socioeconomic inequalities unjust, this proxy only reinforces such injustices. Moreover, it might be considered insulting because it entails buying one's right to follow one's conscience.

The third option, a lottery, does offer a feasible way to distinguish between persons who should get an exemption and who should not, as this would be reduced to what the lottery decided, but it does not offer any distinction at all between sincere and insincere objections, and that is what the decision procedure should be about. Consequently, it does not take seriously the depth of some people's objections to vaccination. Genuine objectors seek an exemption because they want their convictions to be taken seriously, not because they have won a lottery. So, although a lottery might grant exemptions to some people with deep objections, this method may be deemed so insulting that it will be despised and may therefore even be rejected by people with deep objections.

6.5 Conclusion: The Impossibility of Fair and Feasible Exemption Policies

In this chapter, we argued that to be feasible, *rule-and-exemption* policies need to comply with three requirements simultaneously: the limitation requirement, the justice requirement, and the distinctiveness requirement. The US pre-1971 rule complied with the limitation requirement but not with the justice requirement as we would interpret it nowadays. The European approach that emphasizes the "level of cogency, seriousness, cohesion, and importance" complies with the justice requirement but not with the limitation requirement. The justice requirement cannot be met in such a way that the distinctiveness requirement is satisfied as well: government agencies should be able to *distinguish* between sincere objections to vaccination and so-called exemptions of convenience. The more formal—instead of substantive—the criteria become, the more the distinction between religious and philosophical convictions collapses. That is desirable from the point of view of state neutrality, which must be endorsed in a pluralistic democracy. However, there is a second effect: the more formal the criterion, the harder it is for government agencies to separate genuine claims from plain free riders, endangering the distinctiveness requirement.

We can now conclude that in a liberal democracy, it is hard, maybe even impossible, to combine compulsory or mandatory immunization policies with policies that allow for nonmedical exemptions. To be feasible and justified, exemption policies for childhood vaccination should meet all three requirements simultaneously, and this appears to be impossible. The limitation requirement, limiting the number of exemptions, can only be satisfied when the justice requirement is violated. And complying with the justice requirement undermines the distinctiveness requirement. This implies that many countries (at least almost all states in the US) have immunization policies that are inconsistent with basic democratic principles and generally held objectives of public health. The 2015 legal change in California that abolished all nonmedical exemptions not only is to be applauded, as it has led to a better control of vaccine-preventable diseases, but is also much more in line with basic democratic principles.

Allowing nonmedical exemptions would have been one way to build a more reasonable and proportionate policy on the basis of the principled argument for nonvoluntary vaccination that we developed in the previous chapter. What other options do we have to find an optimal balance between protecting public health and respecting individual liberties?

7   A Framework for a Proportionate Childhood Vaccination Policy

In chapters 4 and 5, we argued that the state has a compelling interest in protecting the basic interests of children by preventing (major) outbreaks of serious vaccine-preventable infectious diseases. The most effective way in which such outbreaks can be precluded is through the maintenance of robust group immunity, and the only way this can be achieved is through mass vaccination. We offered a principled argument for our thesis that a democratic government is justified in imposing liberty-limiting vaccination policies when this is necessary to prevent harm to others. However, this interference in individual freedom should not be disproportionate and more intrusive than necessary. Herd immunity does not require everyone to be immunized. Outbreaks of measles, one of the most contagious infectious diseases, can be contained at a 95 percent immunization coverage and other diseases at an even lower rate. This implies that there is theoretical room to tolerate nonvaccination. If herd immunity is robustly guaranteed, unvaccinated children are protected indirectly.

Given state agencies' responsibility for protecting the basic interests of children, how much leeway can they give to the practice of nonvaccination? One way of providing this leeway is by granting exemptions for parents with religious or "philosophical" objections. However, as we argued in the previous chapter, nonmedical exemptions cannot be justified in a democratic context. A liberal-democratic government must be neutral toward different religions and philosophies of life. Yet this neutrality makes it impossible to set fair and feasible criteria to distinguish between vaccination objections that are embedded in a deeper religious or secular worldview, and therefore should be granted exemption, and objections that do not warrant such exemptions.

In this chapter, we explore a different route toward a reasonable and proportionate application of the harm principle in this context. Sections 7.1 and 7.2 explore the principle of proportionality in more depth. We explain how some of the elements of this principle, notably the idea of the "least intrusive means," are much less straightforward than often assumed. Next, we present the main factors in a vaccination program that can be adapted to shape a proportionate policy. We argue that these decisions often require a pragmatic approach, that also takes historical, epidemiological, and cultural contexts into account. At the end of the chapter, we present our view on the contours of a proportionate mandatory policy.

7.1 Taking Context Seriously: The Expediencies of the Case

Even though the harm principle offers a strong and principled ground for the introduction of liberty-limiting measures, it depends on specific circumstances whether, when, and which form of coercion is actually justified. This is consistent with John Stuart Mill's own understanding of the harm principle. He argued that, even if liberty-limiting measures will prevent harm to others, there may still be good reasons not to implement them:

> But these reasons must arise from the special expediencies of the case: either because it is a kind of case in which [a person] is on the whole likely to act better, when left to his own discretion, than when controlled in any way in which society have it in their power to control him; or because the attempt to exercise control would produce other evils, greater than those which it would prevent. (Mill, 1991, p. 16)

Mill mentions this in the context of policies that require us to behave in a particular way—to *do* certain acts and not just (negatively) refrain from engaging in certain harmful behavior—as is the case with contributing to a public good like herd protection.

So, what could be the sort of reasons arising "from the special expediencies of the case" that would support forgoing compulsion or force? The second reason that Mill offers is very much in line with his broader utilitarian point of view: whether force is justified depends on how the consequences of using force are to be evaluated and compared with the consequences of allowing the harm to occur. Exercising control by forcing parents to have their children immunized might well lead to all sorts of evils. It could invoke public resistance to vaccination and distrust in government and public health agencies, which in theory could be counterproductive and lead to even lower overall vaccination rates. If children must be vaccinated before they go to school, more and more parents could decide to homeschool their children, which would be disadvantageous for many children because they might receive a substandard education. And if one specific health program, immunization, is mandatory, people may assume that other child health programs that are still voluntary are not very important and can be ignored. Judging whether these risks are real and weighing up the risks of a low vaccination coverage will be important in policy making that concerns mandatory or compulsory immunization.

The first reason that Mill offers for not using force may also be read as a consequentialist concern: if individuals are free to follow their own judgment, this may in effect lead to behavior that is better for all of us. After all, most parents, because they care about the health of their offspring, vaccinate voluntarily and with no hesitation whatsoever. But this also suggests a different and more obvious interpretation of Mill's argument: the introduction of nonvoluntary policies can only be justified if it really is *necessary* to prevent harm. The use of force is *illegitimate* if it is unnecessary to prevent outbreaks, for example, when there are alternative (nonmandatory) policy options that sufficiently protect robust herd protection. The basic gist of this example is as follows. Even if the harm principle applies, implying that there is a principled basis for compulsory or mandatory immunization policies, deciding *which* liberty-limiting policies are justified and thus *how* immunization should be regulated ultimately requires weighing the values of liberty versus the values served by public health and possibly other values relevant in this specific context. Restricting parental prerogative is justified but only if it is in proportion to the value of the health that is to be protected. And this is not a general verdict; it depends, as Mill says, on "the expediencies of the case at hand."

In the next sections, we revisit the legal principle of proportionality as introduced in section 3.9 and develop a framework for the proportionate use of coercion in vaccination policies. Our elaboration of the various elements of proportionality and their application to the case of childhood immunization programs will show how, as Mill says, judgments about what measures are proportionate depend on contextual factors. This implies, among other things, that we need to take a largely pragmatic and contextual approach to answering the following question: what forms of coercion are justified in response to a declining or otherwise suboptimal vaccination rate?

7.2   The Principle of Proportionality Revisited:
Legality and Effectiveness

In section 3.9, we introduced the legal principle of proportionality in the form of a four-pronged test. Fundamental rights can only be legitimately infringed if (1) the policy goal is legitimate, (2) the measure is suitable for achieving that goal, (3) there are no less intrusive policies available that are as effective as this right-infringing measure, and (4) the measure is reasonable, that is, it takes the interests of all involved into account.[1]

We have already discussed the first requirement of legitimacy extensively. In chapter 2, we argued that the protection of society at large and, more specifically, the health of the population is a central task of government and explained how this offers a justification for collective immunization programs. In chapter 4, we presented our principled argument that maintaining group immunity is a legitimate task for the state: it fits well in the scope of the harm principle and hence is a legitimate basis for interfering with individual liberty. In chapter 5, we discussed the state's responsibility to protect children whose parents refuse to have them vaccinated. Although it is the parents who determine what is best for their children, it is ultimately the government's responsibility to secure a child's basic interests. In exceptional cases, this justifies enforcing immunization against the will of parents—to protect a child from an infectious disease. But outside the context of disease outbreaks, the most appropriate way to protect this basic interest is by maintaining group immunity.

However, policies that embrace more coercive measures to maintain robust group immunity should also be effective in achieving this goal, which is the second condition of proportionality. Ideally, there would be evidence that such a policy will be effective and not backfire during the attempt to achieve the goal. Recent studies on vaccination policies in Europe show that countries that introduced mandatory programs in the past have significantly higher immunization rates and a lower incidence of diseases like measles (Vaz et al., 2020). Yet what we need is not evidence about correlations between types of policies and vaccination rates, as the latter can be determined by all kinds of cultural, political, and historical factors, but evidence about the positive effects of policy change (Attwell et al., 2018; Colgrove & Lowin, 2016). Do more coercive measures result in higher vaccine coverage? Such evidence is inevitably limited, and often the best proof available is knowledge about how specific novel policies have worked out in other countries. But again, there can be large differences in factors that are relevant to policy effectiveness: differences in disease epidemiology and in cultural background affecting people's willingness to comply with laws, the nature and magnitude of sanctions, the number of parents who have refused to participate in the immunization program so far, and the level of trust citizens have in public health authorities. That said, in all recent cases where governments decided to implement more strict policies, this resulted in significantly higher coverage. For example, in Italy, within twenty-four months of extended mandatory vaccination, the coverage rates for the mandated vaccines increased between 3 percent and 7 percent. With regard to measles, the required coverage rate of 95 percent was almost reached within two years (D'Ancona et al., 2019). Similar positive effects were seen in France (Lévy-Bruhl et al., 2019), California and other states in the US (Richwine & Avi Dor, 2019), and Australia. Predicting the impact of policy change will always be difficult, but at least recent experiences in countries that enacted more strict vaccination mandates do not offer grounds for concern that implementing more coercive policies will be counterproductive or not have the desired effect.

For now, we can conclude that the first two conditions for proportionate coercive immunization, legitimacy and effectiveness, can be met. Which types of measures exactly will be effective and how effective these will be differs between countries and depends on many contextual factors. Cultural, historical, and epidemiological context will be even more relevant if we turn to the other two conditions: subsidiarity and fair balance.

7.3   The Principle of Proportionality Revisited: Least Intrusive Means and Fair Balance

At first sight, the third condition of least intrusiveness seems to be much more straightforward than the fourth condition of a fair balance of interests. Determining which measure is least intrusive only requires ranking the different interventions in terms of the extent to which these interfere with fundamental rights, and that assessment seems relatively uncontroversial. Fair balance, on the other hand, requires finding a correct equilibrium "between the demands of the general interest of the community and the require-ments of the protection of the individual's fundamental rights."[2] A norma-tive judgment must be made about how the degree of intrusiveness—hence the value of liberty—weighs against the importance of societal protection against specific infectious diseases. Is the level of intrusiveness of a measure reasonable and proportionate given the magnitude of the desired effects it is meant to have, taking the interests of all those affected into account? In this subsection, we elaborate on the conditions of least intrusiveness (or subsid-iarity in law) and fair balance, arguing that the former is not as simple and uncontroversial as it seems and that both criteria are closely connected and require a contextual and pragmatic judgment.

The principle of the least intrusive means is well established in law and ethics, especially in public health ethics. The core idea is that more restric-tive measures cannot be justified if there are less restrictive alternatives that have not been tried or considered. The Nuffield Council on Bioethics elab-orated this principle by presenting what it calls "the intervention ladder," which ranks a variety of health policies, starting with completely voluntary measures (e.g., offering health information), proceeding to more coercive approaches, and culminating in the extreme case of enforcing specific behav-ior (Nuffield Council on Bioethics, 2007). Our own table of policy options, as presented in box 2.1, repeated here as box 7.1, can be considered an interven-tion ladder applied to vaccination policies. We have not included the specific option of allowing nonmedical exemptions in this table, as we have argued in chapter 6 that such policies cannot be justified in a liberal democracy.

In theory, applying the principle of the least intrusive measure simply requires such a ranking of alternative policy options in terms of how far they impose limits on freedom. The next step is to assess which options suffice to attain the aims of the policy—in our case, to achieve robust herd protection—and then to choose the option within that subset that is least intrusive. There are, however, some complications and even flaws in this line of reasoning, and these can only be solved by taking a broader approach to weighing the competing values at stake.

A first practical problem is that ranking policy options in terms of intru-siveness can be rather difficult (Dawson, 2016). Is requiring vaccination as a necessary condition for (financial) child benefits less intrusive than requir-ing it for school entry if parents can also be exempted in the latter case? Arguably, such measures will impact different parents differently, depending

Box 7.1
Degrees of Coercion in Vaccination Policies (Repeated)

Voluntary policies: encouraging

information campaigns
offer vaccinations free of charge, easy to access, adequate reminders
persuasive communication; positive nudges
offer opportunities for persons not vaccinated in their youth to catch up
allow child day care centers or schools to publish vaccination rates

Voluntary policies: norm expressing

strong nudges, such as making vaccination a default choice option
require child day care centers or schools to publish vaccination rates
opt-out policy: parents must take action if they choose to avoid vaccination
allow child day care centers and schools to refuse unvaccinated children
expand possibilities for lawsuits in case someone is infected by an unvaccinated person

Mandatory policies

set vaccination as a condition for child benefits
require that all children attending child day care centers are vaccinated
require that all children attending schools are vaccinated

Compulsory policies

require that all children in schools are vaccinated, without exemptions, and back this up with financial penalties
make vaccine refusal a criminal offense with punitive sanctions

Enforced vaccination

impose vaccination with force (i.e., against the will of a person or their parent)

on their socioeconomic position. What is experienced as very intrusive by some parents may have hardly any impact on others. This triggers a more fundamental problem. The intervention ladder looks at the extent to which policies respect liberty. But as presented, the tool merely looks at negative liberty and not at positive freedom. It may well be that policies that are more restrictive can at the same time strengthen people's capabilities, putting them in a position that enables them to make choices that are more in line with what they value most. For example, some Dutch orthodox reformed denominations fiercely oppose childhood vaccination but also accept the power of the state as the worldly envoy of God.[3] Devout parents who are inclined to follow religious prescriptions but are very nervous about the possible negative health impact might be relieved when the state legally enforces vaccination, absolving them from the responsibility of making the decision themselves. Parents leaning toward vaccination but hesitant because their religious leaders object to it may in fact be liberated if the state legally compels them to participate in the program. The same applies to parents who cannot make sense of the conflicting information they are confronted with about the possible benefits and alleged risks of immunization. If liberty is a central value, both positive and negative liberty need to be taken into account, yielding a more complete picture that cannot be captured in a one-dimensional ladder (Byskov, 2019). Mark Navin and Katie Attwell argue that this discussion, primarily revolving around parental autonomy versus the value of community protection against disease, disregards the plurality of the moral values at stake (Navin & Attwell, 2019).

A second problem is that more intrusive measures, rather than only the "least intrusive alternative," often need to be considered as well, as a matter of precaution. Policy choices are made in the face of uncertainty about how herd immunity will develop over time and about possible future outbreaks. Policies also need to be decided for a longer period—they cannot be adjusted on a day-to-day or even year-to-year basis. To create robust protection against infectious diseases in the long run, policies might well need to be more "intrusive" than strictly necessary for the foreseeable future.

This makes it clear that which measure is "least intrusive" cannot be decided solely by comparing the intrusiveness of alternatives. It also involves weighing short-term and long-term perspectives; competing interests and values, including positive and negative liberties; and the protection of individual and public health and societal welfare. Judgments about what is least intrusive and which policy strikes a fair balance between competing interests and values cannot and should not be separated. Such a balancing exercise can also not be done in an abstract way: the proportionality of measures needed to promote immunization will depend on a variety of contextual factors that may well differ in different countries, times, and circumstances and with respect to different features of specific infectious diseases. The requirement to have children vaccinated as a condition of being allowed admission to child day care centers is a much more intrusive measure in countries where childcare is necessary for parents to be able to go to work than in countries or cultures where it is common practice and feasible for grandparents or other family members to take care of virtually all young children. Mandatory measures are easier to justify in countries where local outbreaks are more common. And it is more justifiable to introduce mandatory measures to protect citizens against most severe diseases such as measles and polio rather than against somewhat less dangerous conditions like chickenpox.

This brings us to the fourth step in the proportionality test: the measure must be reasonable, considering the competing interests of the people in the relevant society. In this final step, an *all-things-considered* analysis is required that involves weighing the competing claims and values at stake. Even though the narrow proportionality assessment primarily involves weighing the value of (public) health against the importance of protecting liberty rights, it is not a straightforward two-dimensional problem. For one thing, acknowledging the right to freedom of religion of parents can, in certain cases, imply that the right to education of children is constrained. Moreover, it could be that an effective and proportional measure is still unacceptable because it generates unintended negative external effects, for example, through the ways the measure is implemented. For instance, what if a more coercive measure raises the vaccination rate in the short term but at the same time lowers the long-term confidence in vaccination programs or generates much polarization in society between supporters and opponents? Or what if mandatory vaccination to access childcare blocks parents (usually mothers) from entering or remaining in the workforce or implies that the state is no longer able to monitor or supervise unvaccinated children, simply because they move out of sight (Navin & Attwell, 2019, p. 1045)? The possibility and potential impact of such unintended external effects should be included in the proportionality considerations.

In conclusion: determining whether an immunization policy is justified cannot be done in a theoretical vacuum. It requires the assessment and weighing of many different contextual factors: the context and the severity of diseases, epidemiology, the efficacy of the vaccine, the effectiveness of a particular policy, the strength of societal institutions, and the social and cultural background. Most important—and this brings us back to the idea behind the principle of the least restrictive alternative—it will depend on the extent to which it is possible to maintain a high level of group protection based on voluntary participation only.

7.4   A Regulative Framework for Immunization Policies

Judgments about the proportionality of policies aiming to ensure high participation should be context dependent, and this renders it impossible to propose one single set of measures that can be justified universally. It is, however, possible to offer a general framework for assessing the proportionality of more coercive vaccination measures. In this subsection, we present and discuss several aspects of a well-considered immunization policy that involves important choices and explanations. The dimensions of a proportionate policy can be structured along the lines of several questions. Why are liberty-limiting measures taken? How can we limit freedom? When should we do so? What vaccines should be mandatory? And how long should mandates remain in place?[4] The general answers to the first question will not be different for different democratic contexts, but the answers to all the other questions could offer various ways in which policy can strike a balance between the competing values at stake, taking the specific cultural, societal, and epidemiological contexts into account. In this way, the framework offers room for different immunization policies in different societal and political contexts and cultures but only, of course, within the limits of the liberal-democratic principles on which our framework is based.

7.4.1   Why? The Justification of Coercive Measures

Vaccination policies can only be proportionate if they are based on and fit within relevant legal and moral principles that shape constitutional liberal democracies. In chapters 2–5, we outlined these principles and argued that the protection of fundamental rights is one of these foundational values. We also established that liberal-democratic states have a general responsibility to protect society against (the disruptive effects of) dangerous infectious diseases. This sometimes involves setting limits on fundamental freedoms of individuals in order to curb the spread of the disease. Herd immunity not only makes it almost impossible for people to infect one another but is also the most appropriate route for the state to meet another responsibility: protecting the basic interests of young children when parents decide not to immunize them. These principled grounds do not determine the precise character of a liberty-limiting immunization policy; they leave open a variety of possibilities for interventions that may or may not be proportionate, depending on contextual factors. It will be intuitively clear that a policy that compels parents to vaccinate their child against a relatively innocent disease like chickenpox by threatening them with an imprisonment is disproportionate. At the same time, some forms of legal coercion can be justified as protection against more serious diseases. Next, we review in more detail the main dimensions of how programs can be more or less coercive.

7.4.2 How? The Character of Measures

Voluntary policies Arguably, when considering the justification of coercive measures to promote vaccine uptake, little needs to be said about *voluntary policies* that aim to encourage vaccination. It is, however, important to be aware of the various noncoercive options for two reasons. First, it is obviously desirable to enable voluntary choice—not only because of the costs of coercion but also because this acknowledges the moral value of the motive people will have: to protect their own child or to altruistically contribute to the protection of others (Kraaijeveld, 2020).

Second, the introduction of mandatory policies is only proportionate when it is necessitated by (the threat of) an undermined herd immunity. This implies that the state has the obligation to perform to the best of its ability to preclude the necessity of mandatory measures. It should do this by employing all reasonable measures it has available to encourage and accommodate voluntary vaccination.[5] The bare minimum is, obviously, that governmental agencies develop communication strategies to promote vaccination and to actively find ways to reach out to all relevant groups. It should try to understand the reluctance some groups might have toward vaccination and its own (past) role in this vaccine hesitance (Attwell et al., 2022, p. 575). In addition, governmental agencies should enable access to vaccines and their administration and guarantee the availability of a sufficient supply of safe vaccines free of charge to parents or their health insurance company. They should ensure that vaccine services will reach all, including disadvantaged populations, culturally and linguistically diverse groups, and those living in remote regions. We agree with Attwell et al. (2022) when they argue that "it is not enough to just build a resource, such as vaccine information or instructions on how to get vaccinated, in the right language. Resources must also be developed and disseminated in ways that are culturally sensitive and appropriate" (p. 577).

Moreover, governmental agencies should make it as easy as possible for parents to have their children vaccinated by offering vaccinations at convenient locations or during extended opening hours that are adapted to the possibilities of parents of young children. Offering adequate information about how vaccination protects health and countervailing misinformation are also tasks that states should perform.

Additional voluntary policies include measures to protect unvaccinated persons against infections. Public health agencies can actively provide travel advisories to parents about areas in the world where group protection against the relevant diseases is lacking to ensure that unvaccinated children do not encounter such diseases unconsciously. They should maintain up-to-date records of individual vaccination uptake—and the lack thereof—to ensure that everyone has access to their vaccination status later in life. Another possibility is actively approaching young adults aged around fourteen and older to warn them about the risks of not being vaccinated to enable them to catch up on missed vaccinations easily and free of charge. In many jurisdictions, medical treatment can only legally be given to teens with parental consent, so this approach may not help children whose parents have refused immunizations.

If policies are voluntary, it is important that they create a positive incentive. Ideally, participating in a childhood vaccination program is less burdensome than opting out. This is often not the case—not even in mandatory vaccination programs: in some states in the US, getting an exemption used to be less burdensome than having one's children vaccinated. Voluntariness does not imply that the state is bound to employ a hands-off approach or be neutral about the choice parents are making. The Dutch program consists of a comprehensive statewide net of child health centers that entices parents to vaccinate by employing an effective system of vaccination reminders. Parents can ignore the schedule, but the program suggests that vaccination is the norm and calls on parents to comply with the schedule. This brings us to the next category.

Norm-expressing policies   Our next category of policies might still be considered voluntary, but the extent to which they are actually noncoercive depends on societal and cultural factors. The aim of norm-expressing policies is to make it clear that vaccination is the norm, even if it is not enforced. If this norm is not expressed explicitly, the government is communicating that parents have a lot of leeway regarding this issue. People might be less hesitant about getting vaccinated when the government makes clear that everyone has a responsibility to contribute to building protection against diseases like measles to protect their own children and others.

Another example of norm expression is that a state does not impose a legal obligation to vaccinate but explicitly allows nonstate actors to take actions that affect nonvaccinating parents. Day care centers could be allowed—or even required—to publish vaccination rates or be allowed to refuse access to children who do not participate in the national vaccination program. This could generate serious pressure on hesitant or refusing parents and even stigmatize them. Such stigmatization may or may not be morally justified (Bayer, 2008), but the important thing for now is to acknowledge that societal pressure can be present even without formal coercive laws. A drawback of some of these policy options is that they shift responsibility from public to private institutions, leaving it to them to determine and maintain rules about vaccination. An example of such a norm-expressing policy is a recent bill of law in the Netherlands (see box 7.2).[6]

A less stigmatizing form of norm expression would be an opt-out system that assumes that all children without a medical exemption will have the vaccination unless parents take explicit steps to opt out, for example, through formal notification. Again, this measure quite explicitly communicates that vaccination is the norm. Although parents must explicitly formulate and communicate their choice not to vaccinate, stigmatization is avoided because their choice does not have to be public. Such strong nudges may raise ethical questions, but in this specific context, there are good reasons to assume they are justified (Navin & Largent, 2017). On the other hand, there is no obvious way of creating a choice situation that makes immunization the default choice and in which it is up to refusers to take specific steps to avoid vaccination. One possibility is for health professionals to visit homes to vaccinate children and discuss other preventive child health options, with parents having the possibility, on the spot, to opt out and justify their choice. Such an outreach approach might have many additional benefits, but it would involve vast investment.

Box 7.2
Norm Expression: Dutch Bill Allowing Childcare Centers to Refuse
Nonvaccinated Children

In 2019, the Dutch parliament adopted a bill of law that would allow child
day care centers to require participation in the national immunization program as an entry requirement. According to the initiator, liberal member of
parliament Rens Raemakers, the bill primarily aims to create informed choice
for parents, enabling them to choose a center that is well protected against
outbreaks of measles. Yet, even though this law promotes freedom of choice,
such a law is far from neutral. By allowing day care centers to refuse unvaccinated children, it expresses and reinforces (but does not enforce) a social norm
that parents should accept immunization.

The bill was criticized by many, including the Council of State, the Dutch
advisory body on legislation, and us (Evers et al., 2019; Pierik & Verweij, 2018,
2019a, 2019b). Apart from being criticized for specific legal problems (freedom
of choice was not considered a legitimate ground for the unequal treatment of
nonvaccinating parents), it was criticized for not directly aiming at the heart
of the problem—namely, the need to promote higher immunization rates.
Notwithstanding the critique, the bill was accepted in the Tweede Kamer (Second Chamber of Parliament), although some parties that voted in favor of it
only did so because they perceived it as a first step toward a more stringent
policy. In 2023 however, the Senate (First Chamber of Parliament) rejected the
bill, so in the end it was not enacted.

Mandatory childhood vaccination programs   Policies that involve *mandatory vaccination* are quite common in many countries. We defined mandatory
programs as state policies that involve withholding valuable social goods
or services from persons who choose to forgo vaccination for themselves
of their children for nonmedical reasons. The most important examples are
policies that make participation in vaccination programs a legal prerequisite
for day care or school attendance. Although there is no federal regulation,
all US states legally require the vaccination of children prior to school or day
care entry. In most states, parents can receive a waiver if they have religious
or philosophical objections. Similar policies have been introduced in France:
from 2018 onward, unvaccinated children have been refused admission to
day care centers, schools, and summer camps. These policies give parents
a choice, but a decision to forgo immunization has serious implications for

parents. Not having access to childcare arrangements or having to arrange home schooling might hamper work–life balance, especially for single parents and two-income households. The freedom to refuse vaccination is severely limited if immunization is necessary for school entry: primary education itself is compulsory in basically all liberal democracies. Hence, freedom to refrain from vaccinating one's children then depends on the possibilities for homeschooling and the extent to which parents can satisfy educational quality requirements that are imposed on homeschooling. If the standards for homeschooling are very high, the freedom to refuse vaccination is minimal.

A disadvantage of policies that make vaccination *only* mandatory for primary school entry, around the age of four, is that this obligation will come rather late for children whose parents decide to postpone vaccination for as long as possible. Since most vaccines are administered in the first eighteen months of a child's life, such an approach could imply that many infants and toddlers remain unprotected for several years. So, although this policy option involves a high level of coercion, at the same time, it allows parents a few years to hold off vaccination, creating room for measles, pertussis, or meningococcal infections. More important, since access to education itself is also a basic interest of children, this policy can also backfire. To the extent that the rationale for mandatory childhood vaccination programs is the protection of the basic interests of the child, linking it to school entry implies sacrificing access to one basic interest in order to incentivize another. Mandatory vaccination to promote herd immunity only contributes to a child's basic interests indirectly, whereas having no access to a basic education undermines a child's basic interests directly. This makes it clear that the relevant considerations and principles in this discussion are not limited to the fundamental right of parents to freedom of thought, conscience, and religion and the societal interest of preventing infectious diseases. The right of children to an education can sometimes play a decisive role in these discussions.

A more promising alternative is to make participation in the national immunization program a legal requirement for child day care entry.[7] Access to day care as the target of this policy has two advantages over access to school entry. First, children attend such day care facilities in the period when most vaccinations are administered, so parents will be directly confronted with the negative impact of their choice not to have their infants immunized. Second, unlike school attendance, that at child day care is not compulsory, and having no access to it does not adversely affect the basic interests of children.[8] This option therefore leaves much more freedom to parents with genuine objections to vaccination. Unlike compulsory policies, which will be discussed below, this closes the door to childcare options for them. Moreover, the main target of these policies is not primarily the small percentage of parents who have already made up their mind, because it is unlikely that this policy will persuade them. Instead, the main target is the much larger group of parents still on the fence. Such parents may have unarticulated doubts based on half-hearted objections, and since they are never forced to genuinely elaborate their doubts, they might continue to postpone making a decision. And as the proverb goes, one of these days is none of these days. If such parents are not compelled by some external trigger to make a decision, they might never decide, and the child remains unvaccinated. If their lack of decision-making cuts off access to childcare, many parents with less articulated objections might reconsider their initial reluctance.

In this way, policies that link vaccination to day care access can effectively harvest this low-hanging fruit and might be sufficient to achieve or maintain herd immunity. This policy option will be especially effective in promoting vaccine coverage in societies in which most parents take their young children to day care, and in such a context, it may well be the middle ground between almost compulsory policies—linked to school access—and genuinely voluntary policies.

Another mandatory approach involves governments making access to child-related advantages, including child allowances, dependent on vaccinations. An example of this is the *no jab no play* plan and the *no jab no pay* plan, as described in chapter 2 (section 2.4.3). The policy allows parents to forgo vaccination for their children, but parents who do not fully immunize their children (up to nineteen years of age) will cease to be eligible for various forms of financial assistance. The strength of this financial incentive depends on the level of child benefits that a family is entitled to. The Netherlands does not have a *no jab no play* policy or a *no jab no pay* policy, but if the country adopted Australia's policy, then the cumulative sum of child benefits that refusing parents of an eighteen-year-old child would have lost would be around €20,000. Of course, financial penalties in criminal law constitute a similar type of incentive, but strictly speaking, *no jab no pay* is not a legal *penalty* but does mean missing out on financial assistance. If parents opt out of vaccination, they cannot enter the child benefit system. It is rather disturbing that (affluent) parents would have the option to "pay a fee" to avoid vaccinations as an alternative to contributing to the common good to protect children. This is even more questionable given that their choice poses a threat to other children as well as their own. The alternative mandatory options appear more logical and appropriate: if vaccination is linked to childcare entry, the negative implication of vaccine refusal is more clearly connected to the aim of the policy, which is promoting vaccination and preventing outbreaks. Linking vaccination to reduced access to child-related advantages goes against the principle of purpose binding in lawmaking. This is because the purpose for which the benefits are intended, supporting parents in their endeavor to raise their children, is quite different from the purpose for which they are reduced or withheld—increasing the vaccination rate. Introducing such a measure could go against a central principle of the rule of law, *détournement de pouvoir*, the misuse of power by the state.

Most parents will understand that outbreaks of infectious diseases should especially be prevented in day care centers and schools. Mandatory policies that focus on day care entry are therefore more explicitly on target. Such policies can also reduce parents' concerns that their child might be exposed to diseases like measles at their kindergarten. For these reasons, policies related to day care entry—possibly extended to school entry if necessary— are preferable to a *no jab no pay* approach.

Compulsory childhood vaccination programs If mandatory policies are still insufficient to attain or restore robust herd immunity, a further step could be compulsory policies: a legal duty to vaccinate, the refusal of which would imply breaking criminal or administrative law and running the risk of punitive action imposed by the government. A punitive action consisting of a fine is not to be considered a fee in exchange for the freedom to make one's own choice about immunization, as in the *no jab no pay* approach. Refusing vaccination means that parents can be prosecuted, convicted, and punished, possibly ending up with a criminal record. Belgium sets an example: parents who do not let their child be vaccinated against poliomyelitis can be punished with a fine or even imprisonment. In recent years, several such couples have been convicted and were required to pay fines of €500 to €1,000. Interestingly, these amounts are much lower than fines imposed by a mandatory *no jab no play* policy and a *no jab no pay* policy. So although legal compulsion is in principle a more coercive instrument, from a financial perspective, it may be experienced by parents as less coercive. On the other hand, the social costs of having a criminal record can be very high. Vaccine refusers cannot "be members in good standing of the political community" but are convicted persons, "since they fail to perform an unescapable legal obligation" (Navin & Attwell, 2019, p. 1047). In some countries, just having a criminal record (irrespective of its contents) may be sufficient to be excluded from certain jobs or official functions. A criminal record can thus be a lifelong stigma.

A possible advantage of the unequivocal message of a legal obligation is that it could make hesitant parents less susceptible to endorsing information provided by denialists: such information gets tainted since it incites parents to illegal behavior.[9]

Enforced childhood vaccination   The most extreme form of coercion is vaccination being enforced: a child is simply vaccinated against the wish of the parents. This bypasses parental discretion completely: deviant parental choices are not just burdened or punished; they are eliminated. An example of this is the 1990 measles outbreak in the US city of Philadelphia that centered on two fundamentalist churches, Faith Tabernacle and First-Century Gospel, whose members do not believe in vaccination—or in modern medicine in general. Nine children died of measles during the outbreak. Ultimately, a court ordered that all the church members' children had to be vaccinated, setting parental objections aside. The judges came to this decision because the children were in direct danger of falling ill and becoming vectors in the further spread of the disease—a risk that can be reduced with vaccination, even after exposure (Rubenstein Reiss & Weithorn, 2015, pp. 967–968).

Forced vaccination seems to be justified only to avert an immediate threat of a dangerous infection. In chapter 5, we outlined the normative basis for such an intervention: the state must protect the basic interests of each individual child, and if these interests are threatened by her parents, intervention is necessary. It is unlikely that vaccination against the explicit decisions of parents could be justified as a means to achieve or maintain herd protection. After all, other less intrusive policies could be chosen for that, including application of criminal law. Criminal law or mandatory policies do not suffice, however, if a particular child faces an immediate risk. In such a case, the child must be protected against their parents, and this involves temporarily preventing parents from having custody, which enables a health professional to administer the vaccination (cf. the discussion of forced blood transfusion in section 5.4).

7.4.3   What? The Content of a National Immunization Program

National immunization programs such as the Dutch Rijksvaccinatieprogramma offer protection against some twelve diseases. Some of them are more infectious and dangerous than others. In this book, we have used measles as the predominant example of a contagious, potentially dangerous infection. The harmful impact of other vaccine-preventable diseases is also beyond dispute—think about diphtheria, polio, and pertussis. Other diseases are less dangerous but can still be serious enough to warrant inclusion of the relevant vaccine in the program. A third set of vaccines is at the time of writing still being discussed for inclusion, for example, the vaccine against varicella, commonly known as chickenpox.

The question of which vaccines are included in a national immunization program is an important one. The more vaccines are included, encompassing vaccines against less severe diseases too, the less the government can simply expect that most parents will just conform and comply with the full schedule. The recent wave of vaccine hesitancy might be an indication that more parents have the feeling that too many shots are given. Including new vaccines in a national program may therefore affect the support for the program as a whole. Even if the assumption of some parents that children receive too many vaccinations cannot be supported by medical evidence, the fact that parents do have such concerns should be taken seriously by public health professionals and governments.

For our purposes, the relevant question is whether, if childhood immunization is mandatory, the coercive measures should apply to all vaccines in the program. The content of such a program is, apart from its liberty-limiting character, another feature that should be taken into account when shaping a vaccination policy in order to make it proportionate. After all, proportionality involves (among others) weighing the value of (public) health and thus the harm to be averted against the importance of protecting freedom. All vaccines in such programs address potentially fatal diseases, but not all are as infectious and dangerous as measles. Does that imply that not all of them may warrant a mandatory or compulsory approach?

Box 7.3
Why Varicella Was Not Introduced into the Dutch Childhood Immunization Program

In 2020, the Dutch government decided to not include immunization against varicella in the program. The most important consideration in the advice of the Health Council was "that vaccination against chickenpox does not currently serve an urgent public health interest in the Netherlands" (Gezondheidsraad, 2020). This lack of urgency can be explained as follows. The epidemiology in the Netherlands is such that the disease is so prevalent that over 95 percent of children have contracted the disease before the age of five. For almost all children, the infection occurs without complications. This has the positive side effect that infection later in life, which is often more severe, becomes very rare. Most children encounter the disease at an age at which it is relatively harmless.

The introduction of the varicella vaccination into the program could ultimately lead to a decrease in both chickenpox and shingles. But successful varicella vaccination would require a sustained very high vaccination rate to prevent the remaining unvaccinated population being infected at a later stage in life, which would cause a higher burden of disease. Achieving such a high vaccination rate was deemed unlikely, and neither public health professionals nor parents considered the health problem of chickenpox to be very important or pressing (van Lier et al., 2016; van Lier et al., 2019, p. 47). Including the varicella vaccination in the program would therefore protect the vaccinated children against the mild form of the disease, but it would probably cause an increased risk for children of nonvaccinating parents (Pierik, 2020a); for the context of the debate, see the work of Malm and Navin (2020a, 2020b).

The health benefits of preventing a serious infectious disease are determined by what the disease means for patients: how severe is the illness, and what is the likelihood of getting infected and falling ill? Arguably, states should only impose prevention with force if this can help avert infectious diseases that may threaten life or may lead to permanent disability or suffering. These risks are also determined by the availability of adequate and timely therapeutic responses to infection or the lack thereof. Moreover, coercion is more easily justified in cases where the chance of being exposed to infection is high and disease can spread rapidly, so it can easily lead to an outbreak that seriously disrupts social life.

A special case is the tetanus vaccine. Spores of tetanus bacteria are everywhere in the environment, including in soil, and these spores develop into

---

Box 7.4

HPV Vaccination of Girls and Boys

Another interesting case is the vaccine against the sexually transmittable human papillomavirus (HPV). Immunization against HPV offers protection against cervical cancer. Should this vaccine be part of the mandatory childhood immunization program?

There are strong grounds to offer HPV immunization to all girls (cf. section 2.3), but mandating this vaccine is questionable. First, HPV does not lead to sudden outbreaks that disrupt society, because the related cancers do not manifest themselves in waves but in individual, unconnected instances (see below). Second, the link with childcare or primary school entry is not relevant due to the age of the children but also because these are not the places where the infection will spread. Second, unless boys are vaccinated as well, it will be difficult to attain and maintain herd immunity, so parental refusal does not clearly undermine the public good. Refusal is of course disadvantageous for the individual girl, but she will be able to make her own choice—though probably a few years later—against her parents' will and be protected in time. Several countries, including the Netherlands, have decided to offer HPV vaccination to boys too so that herd protection is achievable. Would it make sense, then, to mandate it after all? Of course, our first counterargument (the missing link with childcare and school entry) still applies.

Moreover, the special nature of sexual intimacy might be an extra ground for hoping that boys would want to be vaccinated for altruistic reasons. For a more extensive discussion of HPV vaccination for boys, see Kraaijeveld (2020).

---

bacteria when they enter the body. Tetanus does not spread from one person to another. Consequently, there is no such thing as herd protection against tetanus. One can reasonably argue that every individual child should receive protection against tetanus as a matter of equitable access to health and health care, as we argued in section 2.3. The vaccine against tetanus is normally administered as part of a vaccine that protects against multiple diseases, including polio and diphtheria. In the 2021 Vavřička case, the European Court concluded that since every child needs individual protection against tetanus and herd immunity is not achievable, "domestic authorities may reasonably introduce a [mandatory] vaccination policy in order to achieve an appropriate level of protection against serious diseases" ("Vavřička," 2021, p. 65, ¶288). This does not imply that member states are required to offer it through a mandatory scheme, but they are also not prohibited from doing so.

Indeed, more and more vaccinations involve cocktails that protect against multiple diseases, and this has been a major contribution to the success and health impact of immunization programs. In our view, all common combination vaccinations offer protection against at least one disease that is serious enough to warrant a mandatory or compulsory approach: MMR covers measles, and DPPT includes polio, diphtheria, and whooping cough. Distinguishing between mandatory and nonmandatory vaccines would only make sense regarding vaccines that are administered separately, such as vaccinations against HPV, rotavirus, varicella, or meningococcal disease (although even these vaccines often protect against multiple strains of the same pathogen).

In countries with adequate and accessible health care systems, rotavirus[10] is an interesting case because almost all children are infected and experience temporary and mild disease; a small group of patients, however, have complications, require hospitalization, and may sometimes die because of these "mild" diseases. It is not obvious that these diseases are severe enough on a population level to warrant mandatory immunization. At the same time, the disease comes in waves, which can temporarily overwhelm hospitals' pediatric wards. Judging whether they should be part of the mandatory scheme requires a careful assessment of epidemiology, the course of severe illness, and the peak load it can generate for the health system. But it ultimately involves a value judgment about whether or not to accept risks that are very small on a population level but potentially grave for specific individuals. Given that these are contextual decisions, it is not surprising that different countries will judge these risks differently and that some will consider, for example, mandatory rotavirus vaccination to be proportionate while others will not.

7.4.4   When? The Timing of More Coercive Measures

Populations do not need complete vaccine coverage to be protected, even in the case of the most infectious diseases. And herd immunity is also not an all-or-nothing concept. A 95 percent vaccination rate is sufficient to protect against measles, but a vaccination rate of 85 percent also offers a much better collective protection than a vaccination rate of 70 percent. If it is possible to attain and maintain sufficiently high participation in a voluntary vaccination program, this is to be preferred as a matter of proportionality. This observation raises the question of at what point a voluntary program should transition into a more coercive one. A country like the Netherlands, with a voluntary scheme, has seen the MMR (given at two years of age) participation rate fluctuate between 96.2 percent (2006 cohort) and 92.9 percent (2016 cohort) (van Lier et al., 2021). It should be noted, however, that these are national figures; in some villages or parts of cities, coverage is currently way below 70 percent. The World Health Organization recommends that countries aim for 95 percent as this is seen as the percentage needed to eliminate measles. Is any participation rate below the WHO recommended figure a sufficient circumstance for coercion? Here we must distinguish two rather different policy goals: the role of states when they ratify an international treaty that seeks to eliminate diseases like measles altogether and the role of states to protect their (underaged) citizens.

If this latter question is about the proportionality of policy measures, then a threshold level for justified coercion should depend on the nature of the measures envisioned, with a higher level of coercion only applied when the vaccination rate decreases further. One could imagine successive steps of increasing coercion, with, for example, a mandatory approach being justified if participation drops below 95 percent and compulsory vaccination, making refusal a misdemeanor or crime, being justified if coverage is below 90 percent. Determining such thresholds is, ultimately, a matter of political judgment about what sorts of risks are considered acceptable within one's society.

A policy change that involves exchanging a fully voluntary approach for coercive measures will be a controversial decision requiring political courage. It is often suggested that such a change will provoke a lot of resistance and that it may even be counterproductive as it could spur distrust of public health authorities. Recent examples of policy change (Australia, California, France, Germany) have not led to widespread resistance or uproar, but it is still a concern that should be taken seriously. Introducing mandatory measures might be successful regarding avoiding an imminent outbreak but could simultaneously undermine the diffuse background support for vaccination in general. In our view, it therefore makes sense to make political decisions about the threshold for coercive measures at a time when that threshold has not been met. We believe that implementing coercive measures will be much more feasible and sustainable in the long term if they are not hastily imposed in response to an acute emergency. On the other hand, such discussions will not receive much political support if they are conducted in the context of an unthreatened robustly high vaccination coverage, because the issue will have insufficient urgency on an always crowded political agenda. Instead, such discussions should start at the moment the trend of declining vaccination coverage is clearly visible in the statistics or in surrounding countries. This means that such policies are debated in the context of a concrete trigger and, at the same time, have been prepared and announced well in advance of an acute outbreak. This requires politicians to start discussing the issue before it becomes an acute problem—and civil society to put the issue on the agenda.

Interestingly, societal and subsequent political discussions about the choice of parents to forgo vaccination for their children and about the risks this creates for society at large may themselves lead to a higher immunization uptake. This seems to have been one of the factors contributing to a slightly increased vaccination rate in the Netherlands since 2018 after years of decline, even before new policies were established. Ongoing political and societal debate about nonvoluntary measures may generate some pressure on parents or lead hesitant parents to rethink their opposition and change their minds, thus making the implementation of such measures less necessary—at least for the time being.

7.4.5   Until When? The Reversal of Measures

So far, we have been focusing on the proportionality of coercive measures in response to decreasing vaccine uptake. But what if such measures have been successful for years or decades, resulting in a stable uptake of 95 percent or more; would the principle of proportionately then require that coercive measures should be relieved or lifted?

We tend to think they should not happen. Our stance involves a broader perspective on the principle of proportionality: we not only look at weighing the intrusiveness of the interventions against the graveness of the harm to be prevented but also consider the broader burdens and benefits of policy change.

The first argument against lifting coercive measures that have been successful is the risk that uptake would decrease again. A government that considers abandoning coercive measures to protect herd protection must be sufficiently confident that this policy change will not negatively affect participation rates. From a policy perspective, it would undesirable if such a policy had to be reversed *again*, alternating between implementing and revoking compulsory measures.

A second argument for maintaining mandatory vaccination is one of feasibility. The societal impact of *implementing* a coercive measure is presumably much larger than *revoking* such a policy. Public resistance against imposing measures will be concentrated around the time of the decision-making and implementation, whereas calls to revoke the measures will be spread over a much longer period and arguably will continue during the time that the policies are in place, which may be years. It might also be relevant that many people—even those who had previously opted out of vaccination—will get used to the idea if every child is vaccinated as a matter of law. There is an analogy with seatbelts here (Giubilini & Savulescu, 2019). Arguably, many people have internalized the need to use a seatbelt since they became mandatory in many countries, and one could argue that mandatory seatbelt laws therefore interfere much less with their freedoms than at the time of their initiation. Of course, even if everyone endorses seatbelts, a law that requires us to do so is still an infringement of negative freedom. But few people will experience it as such.

A third argument for maintaining mandatory vaccination is that lawmaking also has a symbolic impact, affecting social norms over time. The introduction of mandatory seatbelt wearing and smoking bans were contested when they were implemented but became more generally (albeit never universally) accepted and, consequently, the implicit "new normal" over time. So, even though we need such legal measures to stop a small minority from smoking, smoking bans are now totally undisputed among the large majority of the population, including most smokers themselves. Indeed, it is rather striking to realize nowadays that in many countries that now have smoking bans, it was considered perfectly normal in the 1970s to smoke on trains and planes and in restaurants and lecture halls. It is possible that mandatory vaccination measures, once implemented, will have a similar effect over time: that even resistance that is very vocal at the start will become a marginal phenomenon over time. But the symbolic function of law has an effect: if the coercive measures are lifted, it sends a message that it is no longer a problem if parents refuse vaccination for their child. It is as if the government is saying, "We are happy with current vaccine coverage and from now on it is OK for a small group to opt out." Voluntary programs should not, however, support vaccine refusal at all—and should not even suggest such support.

We conclude that governments have good reasons to stick to mandatory vaccination policies, even if they have led to a stable and sufficiently high vaccine uptake.

7.5   The Contours of Proportionate Coercive Childhood Vaccination Programs

In chapter 4, we offered a principled justification for imposing coercive measures to protect and maintain a level of vaccine coverage that generates robust herd immunity. To achieve that goal, for example, for measles, the vaccination rate does not have to be 100 percent, so there is some space for leeway and tolerating a limited proportion of vaccination refusals. In chapter 6, we concluded that this space for refusal should not, however, be allocated through nonmedical exemptions, because such an approach cannot satisfy some central requirements that a liberal democracy should set for such policies. In this chapter, we formulated a more compelling method for establishing coercive measures in a proportionate way. Liberty-limiting policies are defensible if and only if they fulfill a legitimate purpose, if they are effective and not more intrusive than necessary, and if the interests of all persons concerned have been taken into account and weighed.

In this chapter, we have argued that vaccination policies aiming at maintaining herd immunity do indeed serve a legitimate goal and also that, especially in the context of childhood vaccination, the rights of parents can be infringed legitimately when this is necessary to protect and maintain herd protection. And even though there is a myriad of options for voluntary measures to promote vaccination, such policies may not secure a sufficiently high vaccination rate in all circumstances. The drop in the vaccination coverage after the publication of Wakefield's article that falsely linked vaccination to autism is a case in point here. With this in mind, it is reasonable for governments to consider how vaccination policies can be coercive, yet in a proportionate way. We have outlined the factors that should be considered if a government, confronted with inadequate vaccine uptake, is considering making childhood immunization less voluntary. Proportionality can be achieved and shaped in a variety of ways: by adjusting the nature of measures that nudge or even force parents to participate, by deciding on a smaller or a larger package of vaccinations that are mandatory, and by setting thresholds for vaccine uptake that determine when specific coercive measures are to be implemented. Decision-making about which policies are appropriate in a country will have to consider the epidemiological, societal, and cultural contexts, as well as the strength and accessibility of the (clinical) health care facilities of that country. Thus, what might fit well in one country could be inappropriate in another.

At the same time, we have suggested how some measures are less defensible than others. Some norm-expressing policies, notably those that merely *allow* child day care and schools to refuse unvaccinated children, are problematic as they neglect the fact that protection against infectious diseases is first and foremost a responsibility of government and not of private organizations. The government responsibility is much more central in mandatory approaches, and these have been shown to be effective in maintaining herd protection in many jurisdictions. The most common measure is to make vaccination an entry requirement for primary schools and sometimes also child day care centers; an alternative approach is to link it to child benefits. If low vaccination rates necessitate mandatory policies, we have argued in favor of a policy that makes vaccination required for access to child day care. If this does not yet result in a sufficiently high vaccination rate, a next step is to consider vaccination as a requirement for school attendance as well, although it should be done in a way that it does not damage children's basic interest to education. Linking the requirement of vaccination to child benefits is in our view less defensible as it involves the wrong sort of coercion: it makes refusal a legitimate option that parents can decide to "buy." If there is a preference for financial sanctions, it is better to make them a matter of criminal punishment, hence a compulsory measure. This is because criminal law also includes an extremely powerful expressive element: being convicted and forced to pay a fine conveys the notion that vaccination remains a legal obligation, and paying the fine does not take away the wrongness of refusal.

What should be in the mandatory package? We consider several diseases, like polio, measles, diphtheria, pertussis, and meningococcal disease, as obvious targets for mandatory immunization, because these diseases can spread rapidly and lead to permanent disability or death, and the treatment for them is not straightforward. More discussion is possible concerning, for example, rubella, mumps, tetanus, HPV, hepatitis B, and rotavirus, either because the risks of infection and disease may vary in different regions in the world or because other (cultural, social, economic, health care) factors can result in different judgments about the severity of infection and disease. The case of chickenpox (see box 7.3) shows that deciding on the contents of a mandatory vaccination package involves complex scientific and societal judgments in which many different aspects need to be taken into account. Pragmatic considerations will also play a role. Public policies need to be clear and persuasive, and this constrains the extent to which complexity, generated by philosophical subtlety, can be taken into account. For example, it would not be implausible for public health authorities to prefer *one* mandatory package that is offered to all children, instead of distinguishing between some vaccinations that are mandatory and others that are optional. After all, the optional vaccines will also offer important protection for each child, and the contrast with mandatory vaccines may send the wrong message.

A similar pragmatic stance can be taken toward decisions about a threshold for implementing mandatory measures. Epidemiological evidence and modeling can offer limited guidance for deciding what is an absolute minimum level of vaccine uptake. The objective is, of course, robust herd protection. But what level is necessary is not a simple calculation. It will differ for each infectious disease. Moreover, even a 95 percent vaccination rate in a country may not be enough if there are many small local pockets where less than 70 percent of all children participate. Decisions will therefore be based not only on scientific evidence and modeling but also on pragmatic considerations. Public health programs should preferably be clear and simple, as well as easy to explain and justify to the public. If there are ways to avoid resistance and debates in which antivaccination lobbies take a prominent role, public health authorities have good reason to choose those options. Seeking and maintaining public support for vaccination policies may be considered a rather pragmatic aim, but that does not make it less important: it is essential for any program that ultimately depends on the willingness of most parents to participate.

A policy choice that is a little too pragmatic would be to discontinue mandatory vaccination when, after a long period of declining uptake, figures are on the rise again. In our view, this does not fit well with the principle of precaution for two reasons. One is that few countries with voluntary schemes have been able to attain a vaccine uptake that is higher than 95 percent. A second is that coverage is likely to go down again after a period with fewer outbreaks, and then the risks of disease will become high again, leading to new calls for coercive measures. Vaccination policies—and discussions about changing them—should be coherent and well grounded, not ad hoc. The idea of deciding on a threshold for implementing coercive measures can help in this respect.

If the state is to take both the importance of vaccination *and* the intrusiveness of mandatory programs seriously, it makes sense to use the good times of (almost) sufficient or increasing vaccine coverage to maintain or even strengthen public health policies that will be needed for worse times. For example, in the Netherlands, vaccine coverage slightly increased in 2019 and 2020 but was still below the WHO recommended 95 percent. One possible approach would be to set the threshold for mandatory policies somewhat below the current vaccination rate (e.g., at 93 percent) and to gradually push the threshold up if coverage increased further in the coming years, until the WHO recommendation is achieved. In this way, the immunization policy can become more stringent without an immediate implementation of coercive measures. Such an approach would strike an optimum balance between the competing fundamental rights and interests at stake.

7.6 Childhood Vaccination: A Conclusion

In chapter 4, we developed a generic principled justification for coercive immunization policies. This chapter completes a series of discussions in which we apply the Millian argument to childhood immunization (chapter 5) and present a proposal for a proportionate form of mandatory vaccination. The proposal rejects exemption policies (chapter 6) and instead sets a minimum level of vaccine coverage below which it is considered justified to require all children attending day care centers to participate in the national immunization scheme. By discussing the relevant dimensions of a proportionate policy, we offered a range of possibilities to tailor the proposal to different contexts, which may also guide the democratic policy-making process (which is necessary for coercive measures). In the next chapter, we explore how our principled justification may also offer a basis for coercive yet proportionate vaccination programs for adults.

8   Beyond Childhood Vaccination

Before the COVID-19 pandemic emerged in 2020, almost all ethical discussions on the regulation of collective immunization concerned children. Most of the examples and arguments discussed in this book had the same child-centered focus. This is not only to be explained by the fact that it is often children who, due to their relatively "naive" immune system, are especially vulnerable to infectious diseases and that they are therefore the most important target for national programs. From a regulatory perspective, the more important aspect is that they are too young to make their own deliberate decisions on vaccination and that their parents, who are expected to make medical decisions in their name, sometimes decide against it. This creates a dilemma for governments, which have a responsibility to protect the basic interests of children. In the previous chapters, we argued that mandatory childhood vaccination can therefore be justified in specific circumstances. The same argument cannot, however, be simply applied to adults who are capable of observing their own interests. Can coercive vaccination measures aimed at adults be justified at all?

In this chapter, we first explore in general how the arguments we have developed so far for childhood vaccination can also apply to coercive vaccination of adults—which involves exploring relevant differences between policies aimed at children and those aimed at adults (section 8.1). Next, we discuss in detail vaccination policies in the specific context of the SARS-CoV-2 pandemic (sections 8.2–8.4), which, in our view, offers a good illustration of how adult vaccination can be coercive but also how complex this still is. An important dimension of vaccination during a large outbreak is that there will often already be many liberty-limiting measures in place, and against this baseline, it is easier to justify coercive vaccination policies in the context of a pandemic. In section 8.5, we return to the more general level: is coercion also justified outside the context of a pandemic? Finally, in section 8.6, we evaluate the differences between the policies we defended for vaccination for children and adults.

8.1   Coercing Adults to Participate in Collective Vaccination

In the past few decades, the best-known example of collective immunization programs for adults was probably the yearly influenza vaccine. Other examples are those for shingles or pneumococcal disease, but such vaccinations are offered through fully voluntary programs. And before we discuss coercive measures and their possible justification, we should repeat here what we emphasized in section 7.4.2 on childhood vaccination. More coercive measures can only be considered after all reasonable attempts to cater for and support voluntary vaccination have been employed.

Compulsory or mandatory vaccinations are not uncommon, but they are only for traveling abroad or in very specific professional contexts, so are not generally part of national immunization programs. Countries in Africa and South America in which the yellow fever virus is endemic require incoming foreign travelers to be vaccinated against the disease. In specific professions, people are required to be vaccinated during either training or practice. For example, care workers who work with needles and other sharp objects run more risks of encountering hepatitis B, and in addition to the risk of being infected during professional practice, infected professionals also generate a risk of infecting patients. For these reasons, employers are sometimes required to offer hepatitis B vaccination to every employee if they may be exposed to the hepatitis B virus. Employers may also refuse to give unvaccinated health care workers tasks that involve an increased risk of infection and require them do other suitable work—and this can be made a mandatory policy. Hepatitis B vaccination is not mandatory for health professionals in all countries; for example, in the Netherlands, at-risk employees who work in health facilities are free to refuse it but can be required to have an antibody test every three months.

Outside international travel and professional contexts, a coercive policy for the *collective* vaccination of adults is very hard to justify. To understand this, we have to refer back to the fundamental rights discussed in section 3.5, in particular bodily integrity and the freedom of thought, conscience, and religion. In the context of childhood vaccination, the freedom of thought, conscience, and religion—in combination with parental autonomy—is a fundamental liberty that sets a clear though not absolute constraint on coercive childhood vaccination policies. We have shown under which conditions mandatory vaccination of children can be a justified and proportionate infringement on the freedom of parents. Yet this justification was partly based on the state's responsibility to protect the basic interests of children who cannot (yet) take care of their own interests. Parents have the right to organize their lives according to their own basic convictions, and this freedom also extends to their ideas about what is best for their children. Yet this extension is limited if they make decisions that may be harmful for their child—ultimately, this is the harm principle at work. It will be much more difficult to constrain their freedom of thought, conscience, and religion or belief if it concerns vaccination for themselves. This is a first ground for believing that the bar will be much higher for justifying mandatory vaccination of adults.

A second ground for this normative stance is a person's fundamental right to bodily integrity. Vaccination involves invading someone's body, and if this is done without that person's voluntary consent, it is rightly considered to be even more intrusive for that person than other restrictions of liberty, such as restricting their freedom to move or travel. Being able to determine what is happening with and in one's own body is indeed one of the most fundamental rights in the human rights catalogue. A person's choice to refrain from vaccination is a choice they make about their own body and health, and liberal-democratic governments should be extremely cautious about interfering with that right, as a matter of respect for bodily integrity. Mandatory childhood vaccination, as we argued in section 3.6, does not interfere with anybody's right to bodily integrity; it merely interferes with a parent's choice to refuse vaccination *for their child*, and bodily integrity is a matter for which the state has a responsibility and a right as well: to preserve the basic interests of each child. However, coercing adult citizens to accept vaccination certainly does interfere with their bodily integrity.

To summarize: the fundamental liberty of thought, conscience, and religion that is often invoked against compulsory or mandatory childhood immunization policies is even stronger regarding the vaccination of adults. In addition, the right to bodily integrity may be irrelevant for childhood vaccination policies but it is certainly applicable in the context of nonvoluntary immunization of adult citizens.

At the same time, these fundamental liberties of adults, even their right to bodily integrity, can be legitimately constrained by an appeal to the harm principle. In exceptional cases, it is conceivable that vaccination of adults is necessary for the protection of the health of others, and in such cases, the harm principle applies—as explained in chapter 4. If vaccination is necessary to prevent direct harm to others, or, the more plausible case, if maintaining a high vaccination rate is necessary to protect public health and society at large, coercion can, in principle, be justified.

A core element of our justification for childhood immunization was the government's responsibility to protect each and every child's basic interest to life and health. In exceptional cases, this can amount to enforcing vaccination against the will of their parents, but in normal times, it will support proportionate mandatory policies to ensure robust herd immunity against certain vaccine-preventable diseases. One may question whether the state has a similar and far-reaching responsibility to protect each and every adult. It is already clear that the bar for justified coercive policies is much higher in the case of adult immunization. After all, the primary responsibility for their health lies in the hands of these adults themselves.[1]

Nevertheless, the protection of public health may sometimes require coercive policies. There are a few cases when legal force was used, and the aim was the collective immunization of adults to protect the health of others. The 1905 Supreme Court case *Jacobson v. Massachusetts*, about compulsory smallpox vaccination, which targeted all citizens of Boston, is still a landmark verdict in US public health law. More recently, in 2019, the mayor of New York required all inhabitants in several quarters of the city, regardless of their age, to be vaccinated to control a severe measles outbreak. This requirement was backed up with punitive measures that could have involved a $1,000 fine (NYC Health Department, 2019). By mandating the measles vaccination for everyone, children and adults, it was hoped that risks for children too young to be vaccinated themselves would decrease.

It is not only health interests that are at stake, however—especially when infectious diseases are hitting adult populations as well. Indeed, the most evident kind of harm that might justify the restriction of adults' rights results from the societal disruption that emerges during a large-scale outbreak of a new infectious disease and the pressure it puts on the health care system. The

COVID-19 pandemic is a predominant example. In the next sections, we discuss more specific forms of coercive public health policies by taking a closer look at the ways in which the COVID-19 pandemic emerged and the discussions it generated on mandatory and compulsory vaccination of adults.

8.2   The COVID-19 Pandemic and the Societal Disruption It Caused

In December 2019, hospitals in Wuhan, a Chinese city of 11 million inhabitants, saw a rise of cases of lung disease, including pneumonia. After some time, the disease was traced back to a food market where live animals were sold. At the beginning of the outbreak, it was assumed that the disease did not transmit from human to human, but as the infection appeared to spread rapidly, it became clear that this was happening. Within a few weeks, the SARS-CoV-2 virus had generated the COVID-19 pandemic that took the world by surprise.

The nonpharmaceutical pandemic response measures taken from 2020 onward were unprecedented in their magnitude and intrusiveness on individual freedoms. They can only be compared to how measures were implemented during smallpox outbreaks in the nineteenth century (Hirose, 2023, pp. 79–100). Schools, universities, offices, shops, bars, restaurants, gyms, theaters, and cinemas were closed, and festivals were canceled—often for several months. People had to work and study from home, state borders were closed, and some countries introduced curfews. People were only allowed to leave their home for essential reasons and, if they did go out, had to wear protective face masks. Symptomatic patients and those who had been in contact with them were quarantined. Even attendance at funerals was restricted to just a few people. Air travel was banned almost completely, and other restrictions applied to traveling more generally.

The nature and extent of the measures differed between countries: some governments, like those of Sweden and the Netherlands, opted for relatively mild (yet still intrusive) measures, while others, like those of China and New Zealand, were much stricter. In France, the government had a top-down way of implementing compulsory policies, while other states relied less on government force and more on general instructions. Differences can be explained by many factors, including the local mortality rate and the disruptive impact of the control measures, but also cultural differences, the political climate, and, last but not least, the timing of measures: some countries were forced to accept long lockdowns because early precautions and proactive responses had been lacking.

Arguably, the differences between lockdown measures across countries reflected different epidemiological circumstances and also different judgments about what interventions were necessary and proportionate. The diversity in such judgments is not strange given the high level of uncertainty about how the pandemic would evolve and about the effectiveness of the various measures. In all cases, however, there is little reason to doubt which normative idea offers the justificatory basis for control measures: the harm principle. Societies are justified in curtailing individual freedom to prevent harm to others, and during a severe epidemic, this also applies to activities that can reasonably be assumed to facilitate the spread of the virus.

Fortunately, these liberty-limiting lockdown measures did not exhaust possible societal responses to the pandemic. With exceptional speed, SARS-CoV-2 vaccines were developed and approved. The hope was that vaccination would enable societies to abandon lockdowns and other disruptive pandemic response measures. In December 2020, the US Food and Drug Administration issued the first emergency use authorization for the Pfizer-BioNTech vaccine. Several other vaccines were authorized soon afterward—AstraZeneca, Moderna, and Johnson & Johnson—not only in the US but also in most other countries. The vaccines offered strong protection against the most serious disease symptoms. Over time, it also became increasingly evident that even though the vaccines did not guarantee "sterile immunity" (meaning that a vaccinated person cannot infect others; for an explanation, see section 1.7), they did reduce human-to-human transmission significantly, although less so for some later mutations of the coronavirus. Within eighteen months after the onset of the global pandemic, most high-income countries were able to offer vaccines to all citizens who wanted to be vaccinated, first from eighteen years of age and older, later from twelve years of age, and subsequently even for younger children. In these early stages, there was little or no ground for considering policies that would *require* persons to be vaccinated. On the contrary, in the early stages of the rollout, these vaccines were scarce and discussions primarily revolved around which categories of citizens were most vulnerable to the disease and should therefore be given priority access to the first vaccines. At the same time, the issue of coercive immunization was already being widely discussed in the media and put on the agenda by antivaccination groups that advertised their concerns and their rejection of the possible future use of government force.[2]

When the vaccination campaigns started, they were warmly welcomed, and at the beginning, vaccination rates skyrocketed. Over time, however, the increase in vaccination coverage slowly plateaued, and it became clear that the much-desired protection against the virus might not be achieved with an entirely voluntary program. More coercive measures were debated and introduced in an attempt to further increase the vaccination coverage. An important difference between these discussions on COVID-19 vaccination and those on decreasing childhood vaccination rates that emerged around 2015 is that childhood diseases had been mostly under control for decades due to successful vaccination programs. COVID-19 vaccination programs, on the other hand, had to start from scratch, with novel vaccines, and this all happened in the context of a pandemic concerning a new virus to which not only newborn children but the whole population was naive. Moreover, the COVID-19 pandemic had triggered dramatic response and control measures, so when the vaccines became available, individual freedom was already curtailed severely with lockdown measures, mandatory tests, and quarantine and other social distancing measures. As we shall argue, this situation involving already severely limited rights provides the normative baseline against which justification of policies that seek to promote vaccine coverage must be evaluated during *and* after a severe disease outbreak.

8.3 Admission Passes: Pressure on the Unvaccinated

One of the major societal problems in a pandemic is that health care institutions are overwhelmed with very large numbers of patients in immediate need. If the outbreak causes a respiratory disease, one can expect that intensive care units will be flooded with patients and that there will be shortages of mechanical ventilation. Moreover, as hospitals are caring for more and more pandemic patients, other less acute health care will be postponed, which itself will generate more health problems. This is exactly what happened during the COVID-19 pandemic. The most dramatic waves of the pandemic, especially during the winter months, resulted in peaks in COVID-19 hospital admissions that temporarily overwhelmed both regular and intensive health care. Triage protocols were drafted to guide dramatic decisions: which patients should be offered access and at whose expense (Pierik, 2020b; Verweij & Pierik, 2020; Verweij et al., 2020)? In addition, a variety of essential but nonacute health care treatments, including cancer and heart surgeries, were postponed in order to keep enough acute care intensive care beds available, almost always for patients with COVID-19. The COVID-19 peaks generated a large backlog in essential but nonacute care. An important goal of lockdown measures was precisely to prevent this: to mitigate the peaks in the pandemic and thus to ensure continuous access to essential health care services.

By the time vaccines became available, mass immunization was not only seen as providing the best individual protection against infection. It was also considered the best way to relieve the pressure on hospitals and intensive care units, and it promised to enable at least some lifting of lockdown measures and end other physical distancing measures. Vaccination could open the door to returning to prelockdown school, work, and leisure routines. Collective vaccination would thus be the way out, not only for societies at large but also for individuals who, arguably, could be allowed more freedom once they were protected individually by their shots.

In spring 2021, while still in lockdown, Israel was the first country to introduce so-called green passes allowing vaccinated citizens exceptions to the general lockdown rules by giving only them the possibility of visiting nonessential services such as restaurants, fitness centers, and museums. Many other countries followed suit and implemented passes in several guises. European countries developed a joint COVID-19 certificate that would also enable people to travel between countries. The basic gist of these passes was that vaccinated persons, since they were protected individually, could be given more room to resume pre-COVID-19 recreation activities than unvaccinated persons. Given that often a negative COVID-19 test result also offered (temporary) access, we will use the term *protected access pass* to mean a pass for individuals who are considered sufficiently protected against the (transmission of) infection (Brown et al., 2020; Cameron et al., 2021). Over time, two types of passes emerged to regulate access to events or meetings, which can best be described using the German abbreviations 3G and 2G. A 3G policy offers access to persons who are *geimpft* (vaccinated), *genesen* (recovered from COVID-19), or *getestet* (recently tested negative for COVID-19). A 2G policy is more restrictive as it does not provide the option of being *getestet* as a means to get access.[3] 2G policies limit the options of unvaccinated persons considerably more than 3G policies. 3G policies were adopted almost everywhere; 2G policies were implemented in fewer countries. Some governments tightened the restrictions for unvaccinated citizens even further by making vaccination fully compulsory. For example, Austria initiated a law that could punish vaccine refusal with a €3,600 fine every three months.

A follow-up discussion ensued around the *domain* of protected access policies. Should they be implemented only in premises that provide less essential services, such as bars, theaters, or night clubs? Or should they also be implemented in venues that are considered more indispensable: high schools, universities, and police stations? Services are considered nonessential when not participating in or not having access to activities within these sectors or fields has no far-reaching consequences for the person and does not change their legal status as a citizen. The more essential the services for which the passes offered exclusive access, the more the freedoms of unvaccinated persons were curtailed, for example, the right to education in the case of protected access policies in higher education. In some countries, access passes were even required for workers (e.g., in health care or the military), which made it very difficult for unvaccinated people in those domains to hold on to a job. In Latvia, members of parliament who were not able to present proof of COVID-19 vaccination or recovery were excluded from parliamentary buildings, which implied exclusion from meetings and the ability to vote in parliament. Sometimes such limitations were imposed by means of democratically approved national policies; sometimes (e.g., in the US), these policies were also made by private corporations.

Early proposals in the Netherlands about introducing a 3G policy initially triggered vocal political opposition, as it was felt to effectively compel people to accept vaccination. Later on, however, a protected access pass was accepted by parliament, although only for specific nonessential services (Pierik, 2021a; Pierik & Bonten, 2021; Pierik & Verweij, 2020a, 2020b; Verweij & Pierik, 2021). Nevertheless, societal debates about coercive COVID-19 vaccination policies have continued throughout the pandemic, often in a strongly polarized way.

One factor that might have contributed to this polarization was the variety of motives at play for adopting 2G or 3G restrictions. At least initially, governments primarily emphasized that access passes were being introduced to relieve lockdown measures while simultaneously reducing the risk of transmission. If crowded public places were only accessible for persons who were vaccinated, recovered from COVID-19, or had recently tested negatively, this would clearly limit the spread of infection. Such a policy would keep possibly infectious people (unvaccinated, untested) away from places where there is much interaction and risk of transmission. As such, this policy would prevent the chain of infection affecting persons for whom contamination could lead to serious health damage or even death. In contrast, critics of vaccination explicitly emphasized a second possible policy motive, which was less prominent in government communications—namely, that these restrictions were just another indirect measure to pressurize reluctant persons to accept vaccination. Protected access passes did indeed work as an incentive: many countries showed a (temporary) uptick in the number of people booking a vaccination immediately after new protected access policies were announced and introduced.

Over time, the argument that vaccination rates were still too low to contain the pandemic became more emphatically manifest in government communications. The French president, Emmanuel Macron, even went as far as to say that he wanted to annoy the unvaccinated into accepting the shots by squeezing them out of the country's public spaces: "Les non-vaccinés, j'ai très envie de les emmerder! [The unvaccinated, I really want to piss them off!]" (Onishi, 2022). Some countries further tightened the restrictions for unvaccinated groups by switching to 2G.

At the same time, however, it became less evident that even much higher vaccination rates would be sufficient to prevent subsequent outbreaks of the disease: new variants of the virus appeared capable of spreading between vaccinated persons as well. However, even though vaccination did not prevent outbreaks, the vaccines remained highly effective in preventing the severe forms of the disease that ended up as hospitalizations.[4] In public debates, discussants disagreed about which of these arguments for 2G or 3G policies constituted the "real" policy motive, which further fueled the already highly polarized debates.

At the end of the day, it was clear that there was no single silver bullet that would stop COVID-19 infections in a similar way to how a sufficiently high vaccination rate effectively curbs measles, making additional measures unnecessary. COVID-19 vaccines did not provide "sterilizing immunity," and new variants of the virus appeared more contagious and less affected by vaccines, which had been developed for earlier variants. So, even though it was evident that a high vaccination rate was indispensable in curbing and eventually ending the pandemic, it also became increasingly clear that there was no threshold vaccine coverage that alone would protect society robustly against new waves.

Still, outside the peaks of infection, at times of moderate spread, these COVID-19 access pass policies were considered effective in limiting the spread of COVID-19 without necessitating a full lockdown. Moreover, it was assumed, either implicitly or explicitly, that such policies would contribute to the very high vaccination rate that is necessary to ultimately contain the pandemic. For our purpose, the question is as follows: to what extent is the coercion of protected access policies justified? Or should governments implement more straightforward compulsory measures to protect societies against (massive) COVID-19 outbreaks?

8.4   Vaccination during an Epidemic: Restricting Fundamental Rights

In this section, we discuss the justification of epidemic control policies that restrict access to social events or facilities to persons who are unvaccinated. Such policies, which give people who are vaccinated access to social events, fit our definition of a *mandatory vaccination policy*. Earlier, in section 7.4.2, we defined mandatory programs as state policies that involve withholding valuable social goods or services from persons who choose to forgo vaccination for themselves or their children for nonmedical reasons. In childhood immunization policies, this revolves around goods such as access to child day care or child benefits. In the context of an epidemic, protected access passes enable access for certain persons to specific services and events that would otherwise be closed to all as a matter of infection control. An important difference between this pass and mandatory childhood vaccination (apart from the fact that the pass is not about children) is that, as previously explained, this pass will also offer access for individuals who are protected in ways other than vaccination, notably having gained immunity due to a previous infection or having tested negative for infection very recently. The fewer the alternatives to getting access are left, the more the pass will constitute a form of mandatory vaccination.

Can such a semimandatory vaccination policy for adults be justified in the context of a widespread epidemic? Although COVID-19 offers an excellent and dramatic example that we refer to occasionally, in the forthcoming subsections, we present a general normative argument on coercive vaccination policies for adults. We argue that the justification of protected access passes is about more than merely (curtailing) individual freedoms and protecting public health, because protected access policies sometimes have a wider negative impact on society. Our conclusion is that in some cases, *compulsory* vaccination might be ethically preferable to *mandatory* 2G policies.

8.4.1   A Lockdown as a Baseline for Evaluating Protected Access Policies

The context of a widespread epidemic has a major impact on how nonvoluntary vaccination policies should be evaluated. First of all, such policies will ultimately be justified by appealing to the harm principle, and during an epidemic, the risk of severe harm is very real. Hence, such coercive policies will be more easily justified than in epidemiologically "normal" times. Moreover, in cases of severe outbreaks, a range of coercive infection control measures will already be in place. Such measures, ranging from quarantine to social distancing or long lockdowns, also need to be justified (White et al, 2022). They must be necessary to prevent harm caused by infection, the curtailment of rights should be proportionate given the harms to be prevented, and certainly the cure should never be worse than the disease. If mandatory vaccination policies are proposed in such a situation, the obvious route to implementing them is to *release* vaccinated and other non-infectious persons from the liberty-limiting measures that are already in place, for example, via offering these individuals a protected access pass. This makes sense if vaccinated, recently tested, and recovered persons are indeed sufficiently protected against infection and hence against transmitting the pathogen to others.

Interestingly, compared to the baseline of a lockdown, a protected access policy does not constrain people's freedom but enlarges their possibilities for participating in social life. It removes restrictions—at least for vaccinated, recently tested, and recovered persons, who no longer pose a serious risk of further spreading the disease. One might even argue that from an ethical perspective, it is inevitable that these individuals will be granted these freedoms. After all, the lockdown measures should not only be justified in terms of necessity but also satisfy the principle of proportionality. If the risk is negligible that these individuals will be links in the chain of further transmission, it is no longer necessary to keep them in lockdown, and therefore lockdown measures that also apply to them would be a disproportionate infringement of liberty.

In the case of COVID-19, the situation was slightly more complicated. Although immunization did significantly reduce transmission, vaccinated individuals could still transmit the virus to some extent, and therefore it was not obvious that they *should* be released from lockdown. But let us return to the example of vaccines that sufficiently prevent the transmission of a pathogen to curb an outbreak, so that vaccinated individuals play a negligible role in the chain of further transmission.[5] Is different treatment of vaccinated and unvaccinated persons by employing protected access passes justified? Let us discuss the 3G and 2G policies in turn.

8.4.2 3G Policies: Enhancing Freedom, Compared to the Baseline of a Lockdown

Effective 3G protected access policies can be seen as relaxing, in a limited way, the restrictions of a lockdown: they provide more freedom of movement for vaccinated and unvaccinated persons without compromising the goals of infection control. The latter must undergo tests regularly to participate in social life, while those who are vaccinated (or those recovered from infection) have immediate access. Of course, vaccination refusers may experience this as a form of exclusion or as pressure to accept the shots. Yet as long as they have the alternative option of getting tested to get access to social activities without immunization, the 3G policy does not tighten the constraints that were already imposed on them as a matter of infection control.[6] On the contrary, against the baseline of a lockdown already in place, access to events after a negative test also enhances the freedom of unvaccinated persons.

The primary goal and justification for 3G protected access policies is to selectively release society from the most stringent measures without compromising the goals of infection control. They promote vaccination coverage but do not coerce individuals to get vaccinated, since there is still the alternative of taking tests to gain access. This situation changes if the policy is tightened further: if access to testing sites becomes restricted or if the policy changes from 3G to 2G.

8.4.3   2G versus Compulsory Policies

If the policy goal of increasing the vaccination rate in society becomes more important, more intrusive policies may be required. This explains the shift from 3G to 2G protected access policies, which removes the option for unvaccinated persons to employ a negative test as a means to gain access to specific establishments. Under a 2G regime, accepting vaccination becomes virtually inevitable for persons who still want to participate in societal life, so they can reasonably complain that this constitutes a further limitation of their rights.

First, we should be clear, though, about the impact that the introduction of 2G has on unvaccinated persons. Compared to the baseline situation of a lockdown, introducing 2G policies does not change their situation in *absolute* terms. They were in lockdown and remain in lockdown. However, their situation worsens in *relative* terms compared to that of vaccinated persons, because 2G only opens society for the latter. Vaccination refusers who stick with their choice may argue that this policy is discriminatory: they are not treated as equals in society, since they are excluded from social life. Moreover, vaccination refusers can experience 2G policies as a further pressure to accept vaccination, and this limits their right to act in line with their fundamental convictions about how to live (i.e., freedom of thought, etc.). Second, if vaccination is not a voluntary choice, it can be considered an intrusion into their bodily integrity. As a rebuttal, one could argue that if mandatory tests have already been justified under 3G and were accepted by vaccine refusers, mandatory vaccination is not a further infringement of bodily integrity. But this response ignores the fact that most people (certainly vaccine refusers) will consider the injection of a vaccine to be much more invasive than a simple mouth/nose swab.

However, as different as values like equal treatment, freedom of thought, and bodily integrity are, all three complaints can be rebutted by appealing to the same argument that appeals to the harm principle. None of these rights and values are absolute: if the exercise of a right constitutes a genuine risk of harm to others, there can be legitimate grounds for restricting it. Hence, in line with what we have argued throughout this book, there is a principled ground for restricted access policies, especially during a major outbreak during which the lives of many are in danger and societal life is disrupted due to infection control measures. Nevertheless, the bar has to be quite high for a 2G protected access policy not to disproportionately curtail these freedoms.

We discussed the four-pronged proportionality test in sections 7.2 and 7.3. Fundamental rights can only be legitimately infringed by a specific policy if these criteria are met: (1) the goal of the policy is legitimate, (2) the measure is suitable for achieving that goal, (3) there are no less intrusive policies available that are as effective as this right-infringing measure, and (4) the measure is reasonable, that is, it takes the interests of all involved into account.

At first sight, there might be little debate about the first element of proportionality, that the infringement serves a legitimate purpose. During a major outbreak of an infectious disease, few will deny that the protection of public health through containing this outbreak is such a legitimate goal. At the same time, as discussed earlier, we can distinguish two subgoals of protected access policies. First, they aim to enable partly opening up society by loosening the most stringent lockdown measures without compromising the goals of infection control. The second goal is to encourage unvaccinated people to give up their resistance, change their mind, and accept vaccination. This complicates the application of our proportionality test, which, obviously, works best if there is a single straightforward policy goal to be assessed. More often than not, however, policy proposals are more complex, pursuing two or more goals simultaneously, not all of which are always explicitly stated. In our proportionality analysis of the 2G protected access policy, we take both subgoals into account, analyze them separately, and then come to an overall assessment. So let us discuss both goals in turn.

A 2G protected access policy might be (very) suitable for the goal of opening up society without compromising the goals of infection control (criterion 2 above), but it might be disproportionate, given the availability of 3G policies that are less intrusive and might be as effective to achieve this goal (criterion 3). A restricted access policy is clearly more proportional if the spread of the disease can as effectively be contained in a 3G policy in which unvaccinated persons also have the option to get access via a negative test. All in all, we must conclude that a 2G protected access policy, aimed at opening society without compromising the goals of infection control, disproportionally curbs the freedom of unvaccinated persons because a less intrusive alternative is available.

But what if we assess 2G as a means to achieve the second goal of encouraging vaccination? The goal of the policy is again legitimate (criterion 1), there are good reasons to assume that the measure is suitable for achieving this goal (criterion 2), and there might be no less intrusive policies available that are as effective (criterion 3). Still, there are good reasons to conclude that the measure is disproportionate from an *all-things-considered* perspective (criterion 4). In this last step of the proportionality test, we should not only balance the infringement of liberty versus the value of public health but also take all relevant considerations into account and come to an overall assessment of the policy.

What is genuinely problematic in 2G policies regarding increasing the vaccination rate is that the government demands that private actors—restaurants, pubs, museums, sporting facilities—and those who work there must identify unvaccinated people and exclude them from their premises. This just reinforces polarization within society. A 3G policy can be justified during a lockdown because it will (temporarily) exclude *all* categories of persons at increased risk, but a 2G policy specifically identifies and excludes unvaccinated people.

It might be the case that the goal of public health protection by means of promoting vaccination offers sufficient ground for curtailing the freedom of unvaccinated citizens. But not every way of implementing this policy is equally suitable. Achieving this goal is ultimately the responsibility of the state, and law enforcement activities can only be delegated to nonstate actors to a limited extent. This consideration carries more weight the more socially controversial the exclusionary policy is. Checking the vaccinations status of customers is categorically different from checking admission tickets at the entrance hall of a movie theater because the latter task is part of the business process, whereas the former serves an external purpose. Checking the age of a customer before serving a drink in a bar also requires a controlling action by the bartender, but the drinking age of eighteen is a relatively uncontroversial restriction—because it involves minors, for example. Mandatory vaccination, on the other hand, remains a much more controversial policy, and the more controversial the goal, the more obvious it is that government agencies cannot delegate the enforcement of this policy to private actors, especially when a private actor can be criminally prosecuted if they do not comply with this law.

If the primary goal is not so much curbing contagion by excluding unvaccinated persons from risky venues but ensuring that as many people as possible are vaccinated, then government must clearly and explicitly communicate this message in the policy it imposes. And the best, and most honest, way is by making vaccination compulsory for everyone. Noncompliance could be made punishable by a periodical fine that lasts as long as the refuser remains unvaccinated. Such an approach is more straightforward. Government has determined that a high vaccination rate is important to fight a disease but realizes that vaccination is controversial among certain groups in society. In such a situation, government should be very explicit about the aim and address this problem itself directly rather than through the detour of private actors. Moreover, by making refusal illegal, it will also be clear that securing compliance is a responsibility of the government itself—this cannot and should not be delegated to private actors. A 2G policy is disproportionate because it incorrectly puts the responsibility for the enforcement of controversial policies on private actors and thus fuels polarization and undermines solidarity within society.

Bringing the two lines of the proportionality test together, we can conclude that 2G is an unfortunate compromise between 3G and compulsory policies. If the goal is to partly open society without compromising the goals of infection control, 3G is more suitable. If the goal is to increase the vaccination rate, compulsory policies are more appropriate (Verweij & Pierik, 2021). In box 8.1, we show how the same line of reasoning applies to requiring employees to be vaccinated.

It may seem as if 2G protected access policies—one form of mandatory vaccination—are less intrusive and thus more proportional than the compulsory measure of a legal requirement to be vaccinated. This is in line with the Nuffield Council's "intervention ladder": enforceable legal requirements are more intrusive than policies that still leave individuals the possibility of staying home and avoiding vaccination. This view, however, presupposes that the problem is two-dimensional: societal protection through infection control versus the (intrusions into) liberties of the unvaccinated. But taking the wider context into account, especially the fact that 2G policies require private citizens to police others, it becomes clear that other values are at stake as well: these policies undermine social cohesion and solidarity, values that are essential, especially in times of social disruption caused by a pandemic. All in all, we conclude that 2G policies are disproportionate; if it is necessary to coerce adult citizens to accept vaccination, it is much more appropriate and justifiable to make vaccine refusal illegal.[7]

Box 8.1

Can It Be Justified to Require Employees to Be Vaccinated?

Mandatory immunization implies that unvaccinated persons are not allowed access to certain valuable yet nonessential goods. One of the most far-reaching measures in this context is to require persons to get vaccinated as a necessary condition to do their paid work—with the ultimate possibility that they will not be able to get a job (or will lose their job if the requirement has recently been implemented) if they keep refusing. Such a form of mandatory immunization is exceptional because the costs of opting out are so severe that, depending on one's profession, hardly any freedom of choice will be left at all.

There are different possible grounds for requiring employees to be vaccinated. One is that their immunization is implied as part of a broader 3G policy, as discussed in section 8.4.2. If a protected access pass is required for visitors to restaurants, it is inevitable that it will be required for restaurant employees. Such a pass also offers access with a negative test and does not force people to get a vaccine. What about a more straightforward requirement for employees to be vaccinated? This has been discussed especially in relation to health care providers being vaccinated against influenza (van Delden et al., 2008) and, more recently, during the COVID-19 pandemic. For example, in 2021, France made COVID-19 vaccination mandatory for health care workers, who thus risked being fired if they did not comply. The main argument here is that health care providers not only work with vulnerable patients but also have a specific professional duty to prevent infection. Another ground might be that during a disruptive epidemic, it will be essential to prevent too many employees from getting ill as this would put further pressure on an already overburdened health care system. If immunization is necessary to fulfill health care workers' professional duty and to protect health care, such a mandatory policy may be justified.

It is much more doubtful whether it can be justified to mandate immunization for all employees, as the US government did during the COVID-19 crisis. Is such a measure proportionate? If the goal is to prevent infection, then a less restrictive 3G protected access policy could do the job just as well. If the goal is to promote overall vaccination rates, this policy seems rather futile given that it only affects a subset of the population. A compulsory policy that applies to all adults would make much more sense (Pierik & Verhulp 2022).

8.5 Nonvoluntary Policies outside the Context of an Imminent Threat

We argued in the previous section that during a widespread epidemic with severe infection control measures already in place, 3G protected access policies providing more leeway to vaccinated, tested, or recently infected adults are not necessarily liberty-limiting policies. They might actually be a good way to partly reopen society without compromising the goals of infection control. Such protected access policies can only be successfully implemented when vaccination protects adequately against infection, though. However, if such policies are tightened from 3G to 2G to further increase the vaccination rate, compulsory immunization policies are more justifiable than excluding those who are unvaccinated from services or social activities.

This does not settle the question of which of the policy options is most justified after such an outbreak has been largely contained and lockdown measures have been lifted. Can governments continue to impose mandatory or compulsory vaccination on citizens when the threat is no longer present? Before we can answer this question, we need to establish exactly what this immediate threat is about. In countries with a well-functioning health care system, epidemics will especially disrupt society because hospitals (and notably intensive care) are overwhelmed, and dramatic infection control measures may be taken to prevent that. Lockdowns and other social distancing measures are often aimed at "flattening the curve"—to prevent too many patients from being in immediate need of medical treatment at the same time.

When the epidemic is more or less under control, thanks to the fact that enough persons in a society have gained immunity, small outbreaks may still occur sometimes but fade out relatively quickly and thus do not overburden the health system again. However, if individual immunity decreases over time, as is the case with COVID-19, group-level protection may also decline. In that case, to prevent new large outbreaks, it may be necessary to maintain a high level of immunity within the population via regular booster vaccinations. Are mandatory or compulsory vaccination policies justified to prevent a new outbreak even if the threat is not imminent?

In our view, 2G mandatory policies that exclude unvaccinated groups from services or social life cannot be justified. If these are unacceptable *during* a lockdown, as argued earlier, they are even more unacceptable if they are installed *permanently* to *prevent* lockdowns. Hence, if a nonvoluntary approach is justified, it should be a compulsory policy that makes vaccination refusal legally punishable. This will prevent new outbreaks and thus protect public health and undisrupted societal life. If, moreover, a large part of the population shares these aims and is willing to participate, vaccination refusal can be considered harm to others: it obstructs and undermines the joint endeavor to protect all (cf. section 4.3).

Again, whether such a policy can really be justified will be a matter of applying the principle of proportionality. Given that this is about adult persons who are capable and have a right to control their own life and body, the protection of individual liberty and bodily integrity will not be easily outweighed by the values of public health and the protection of society—especially if threats are not imminent. What policy can be proportional? It is impossible to answer this question in general as a full justification will depend on the severity of the disease, the level of infectiousness of the pathogen, and the effectiveness of the vaccine fighting the spread of the disease. A compulsory policy will be more easily justified if there are vulnerable groups who fully depend on group immunity because they cannot secure protection for themselves, for example, because the vaccine is not safe for them or does not provide effective protection. In the theoretical case that everyone could secure their own protection by having booster shots and everyone had optimal access to vaccines and reliable information about the risks and benefits of vaccines, it would be more difficult to justify compulsory immunization. After all, "harm to others" caused by vaccine refusal would then first and foremost affect persons who had opted out of vaccination themselves and who, therefore, voluntarily accepted the risk of falling ill. The harm caused by vaccine refusal is then primarily self-harm, which invalidates the application of the harm principle. However, even in that case there could still be indirect broader societal harm: if the group of (unvaccinated) infected persons who require hospitalization is large, this might overwhelm the health care system, resulting in the postponement of regular health care provision for all patients with dangerous diseases like cancer, metabolic diseases, or heart diseases. In short, the question of whether a compulsory policy is justified cannot be answered in general. But given the fundamental nature of liberty and bodily integrity rights, it would only be justified to maintain a sufficiently high vaccination rate against a disease that is extremely infectious and very dangerous, so that outbreaks do not genuinely overwhelm the health care system.

The next question concerns how to shape a compulsory policy—what room is there to make it as unintrusive as necessary, given that a high but not 100 percent immunity rate would be necessary? Suppose 95 percent immunity in the population would provide a minimum level of protection. At first glance, this seems to create the possibility for booster exemptions of up to 5 percent. However, our argument against exemptions in chapter 6 is equally valid in this context, and moreover, it is difficult to see how exemptions could be legally granted at all if refusal is legally prohibited. A better approach is to "use" the fact that 100 percent immunity is not necessary for individuals who cannot be immunized for medical reasons (medical exemptions), for target groups that are not sufficiently reached by even strong government communication, but also by making the interval between periodic boosters depend on how fast or slow population immunity is waning. The latter would imply that people do not get compulsory boosters more often than necessary for the maintenance of herd protection. Interestingly, although this approach looks very different from our proposal for coercive childhood immunization, the approaches are in certain respects quite similar, as we argue in our concluding section.

8.6 Revisiting Contrasts between Adult and Childhood Immunization

Let us take stock. In the previous chapters, we distinguished mandatory from compulsory policies: the latter imply a legal duty to vaccinate, the refusal of which would imply breaking (criminal or administrative) law and running the risk of punitive action being imposed by government. We have expressed a preference for mandatory childhood immunization policies because these strike a reasonable balance between respect for parental autonomy and the obligation of government to protect the basic interests of all children. Our proposal is to require all children attending nurseries or day care centers to be vaccinated according to the regular immunization schedule but to implement this measure only when vaccine coverage falls below a predetermined threshold level. In this chapter, we have turned our attention to the vaccination of adults, taking the COVID-19 pandemic as an example. We have argued that during a massive outbreak, it can be justified to allow vaccinated persons more freedom than those who are unvaccinated. Just like our proposal for regular childhood immunization, this is a form of mandatory immunization. However, we have also argued that if the goal of the policy is to promote vaccine coverage, rather than to directly prevent transmission during an outbreak, it is ethically preferable to shift policies toward a compulsory approach rather than tightening mandatory approaches that exclude unvaccinated persons from societal life.

To emphasize the coherence of our overall argument, it is helpful to revisit overlaps and explicate some of the contrasts between our different proposals for regulating vaccination of children and adults. First, in both cases, the obvious start is to endorse voluntary programs and ensure optimal access to vaccination, and only if this does not result in a sufficient vaccine coverage should more coercion be considered.

Second, the core of the argument for both proposals is the harm principle. Forgoing participation in a collective immunization schedule can be considered to constitute harm to others in various ways, but the main line of argument is that it obstructs and undermines a collective endeavor to achieve population-level protection. This collective harm offers a principled ground for constraining liberty. In childhood immunization programs, the health (and thereby the basic interests) of young children is especially at stake. In adult vaccination programs, the protection of a well-functioning society plays a much more prominent role.

Third, a key difference is that, in the case of adults, there is a much higher threshold for justified limitation of individual rights, notably freedom of thought, conscience, and religion and the right to bodily integrity. A person's right to make choices in line with their religion or conscience is exceptionally strong if it concerns choices about what happens to their own body—and this is also reflected in the right to bodily integrity. Regarding the vaccination of children, parents' right to the freedom of thought, conscience, and religion—although still important—has less weight, and a child's right to bodily integrity does not have any place at all. The near-absolute character of rights that concern one's own person and body is a ground for seeing coercive vaccination policies aimed at adults as only being justified in exceptional cases, possibly only in the context of a realistic threat of widespread disease or societal disruption due to outbreaks. In the case of endemic childhood diseases, the rights at stake have less weight, and freedom can be constrained more easily—even when there is no immediate threat of massive outbreaks: the maintenance of group-level protection to safeguard the basic interests of all children can be a sufficient ground.

Fourth, this higher threshold for coercive immunization of adults seems to be in tension with our preference for *compulsory* approaches for adults and *mandatory* policies for childhood immunization. One response to this is (a) to acknowledge that, when considered pragmatically, the difference between compulsory and mandatory policies is not as straightforward as it may seem. For parents, the costs of being declined access to (state-sponsored) child day care can be much higher than the costs of a legally imposed fine— it all depends on the magnitude of the sanctions. This response, however, does not explain how it could be proportional to require child day care centers to refuse unvaccinated children, while requiring pubs and museums to refuse unvaccinated adult would be fully unacceptable. What is relevant here is that (b) when evaluating the proportionality of alternative coercive policies (and notably when applying the fourth criterion of the proportionality test), more values are at stake than only freedom and public health. A tightened 2G mandatory policy aimed at adults has a much larger negative societal impact. It excludes citizens from the possibility of being an active member of society and excludes them from specific social activities. In addition, it requires private actors—restaurant owners, sporting club owners—to identify and exclude certain individuals from their establishment. In this respect, this specific tightened mandatory policy aimed at adults leads to much more social exclusion within society than our proposal to require all children who attend child day care to be vaccinated. Moreover, in the latter policy, the determination of the vaccination status of children in childcare facilities is a once-a-year administrative act, while in the former, it requires ongoing checks, day in, day out, at the entrance of pubs, museums, and other facilities. Such a permanent process of citizens verifying the immune status of other citizens distorts societal life and relationships between citizens much more than limited access to child day care does. A *compulsory* policy to maintain sufficient immunity will have, all things considered, a less negative impact on societal life and relations between citizens, all citizens are treated as equals regarding societal activities, and the responsibility to enforce it (by means of a penalty) remains with the government.

Fifth, the previous step shows how we have included a variety of normative and pragmatic considerations in our weighing of the competing values at stake, which is the final criterion of the principle of proportionality. How competing values are balanced also reflects an idea about a just and good society. In both our proposals, we try to establish that vaccine-hesitant or refusing groups are still considered part of the population to be protected—and not as complete outsiders. In the case of childhood immunization, our proposal achieves this by maintaining voluntary policies for as long as possible. For adult vaccination, the preferred policy is such that vaccination refusers are not excluded from societal life.

Unfortunately, antivaccination groups do not just undermine the public good and collective effort of maintaining herd protection by means of their vaccine refusal. They also subvert the collective endeavor by spreading messages that call on everyone not to trust the safety of vaccines ("do your own research!") or the motives of governments and public health agencies ("microchips in COVID-19 vaccines"). If collective trust in vaccination is so important, shouldn't the state also impose constraints on the freedom to spread misinformation, just like they should constrain people's freedom to opt out of vaccination? We turn to that question in the next, penultimate chapter.

9 Toward Trustworthiness in Immunization Policy

9.1 The Challenge of Vaccine Hesitancy

The main argument in the previous chapters consists of two steps. First, liberal-democratic governments have a responsibility to ensure adequately high immunization rates, where possible, to prevent outbreaks of vaccine-preventable infectious diseases. This collective protection is a means to achieving two higher-order goals: the protection of the basic interests of young children and the protection of a well-functioning society—including its economic, health care, and educational institutions—against disruptive outbreaks of vaccine-preventable infectious diseases. In the second step, we argue that acting on this responsibility can imply the use of legal action, particularly the employment of liberty-limiting measures (i.e., mandatory vaccination policies). Such policies can take different forms in different contexts and can involve a variety of measures, constraints, and criteria that ensure the policies are necessary, precautionary, proportionate, and justified.

Ethical problems in public health are often framed in terms of a dilemma concerning the state's responsibility to protect citizens' fundamental health interests versus its obligation to respect the freedoms and rights of all individual citizens. If we conceive the controversy about vaccination only in terms of this two-dimensional dilemma, one could say that our proposed two-staged regulation of vaccination—voluntary when possible and mandatory when necessary—adequately "solves" the ethical problem that many states currently face. This, however, oversimplifies the problem. For one thing, it is mistaken to assume that the protection of public health and the maintenance of herd immunity are solely a task for the state. Rather, it is a collective endeavor of citizens and the state (Verweij & Dawson, 2004, 2007).

Governments can initiate, organize, and promote immunization programs. Ultimately, governments can even initiate policies to make it more difficult for citizens to refuse vaccination. But before more liberty-limiting policies are pursued, governments should seek to convince citizens of the importance of vaccination programs and the benefits and protections these programs offer to individuals and the population at large.

For many people, it is not self-evident to choose for vaccination, and governments and health professionals must create adequate conditions for communication and information to encourage citizens to vaccinate (Conis, 2015). Ultimately, the success of programs is determined by the trust, acceptance, and participation of citizens and their conviction that vaccination is something that is good for their child, for themselves, and for societal life at large. If vaccine acceptance is very low, it is highly questionable whether mandatory or compulsory vaccination would offer a real or sustainable solution. People would look for alternative means for childcare if they were not allowed to access childcare centers, and if too many parents opted out, then using more force would probably be unfeasible. It is also questionable whether coercive measures could receive sufficient democratic support if public acceptance is very low. And if a mandatory policy was in place already, sooner or later a political majority would vote to abandon it. Given that the democratic state depends on its citizen consent to effectively execute policies, it is inappropriate to juxtapose public health and individual freedom as conflicting values.

Moreover, if programs have so far been voluntary but participation rates drop below a certain threshold, political discussion about a mandatory scheme that is to be imposed might only strengthen the opposition to it. Critics could protest that this amounts to the suppression of a minority. Although in various countries, recent policy changes toward more coercive programs did not lead to a drop in the overall level of vaccine acceptance, the possibility of such a backlash cannot be excluded beforehand.

But most important, current vaccine hesitancy and the dilemmas it creates for vaccine policies are not just a matter of judging which value is most important, public health or individual freedom. Even if a proportionate mandatory program *is* widely accepted in society and has broad democratic support, this will not take away or silence the objections of people who object to vaccination or have concerns about the potential side effects. Even though a political majority is convinced that mandatory vaccination policies are, all things considered, fair and justified, the government continues to have an obligation to explain and justify these policies to critics and, indeed, to take their views seriously—even if these are not in line with generally accepted science or expert advice. This is, first and foremost, a matter of respect and good governance, taking seriously the plurality of moral views in a liberal-democratic society. A second, more consequentialist argument for this obligation is that, inevitably, such oppositional voices will keep vaccine hesitancy alive and might spread it further. A democratic government therefore cannot simply push aside epistemic and moral disputes by appealing to the scientific and professional consensus about vaccine safety and effectiveness.

How should governments deal with such opposition toward vaccination, which, on the one hand, can be seen as one of the many voices in an energizing free market of ideas but, on the other hand, can ultimately contribute to an erosion of vaccine acceptance and of state legitimacy in general? We argue that in a democratic context, the state still has obligations toward minorities' points of view that strongly disagree with policies—even if those policies are democratically justified. Although public trust in vaccination is of the utmost importance for democratic governments, the focus should be on making immunization policies and the institutions and professionals that shape these programs *trustworthy*, rather than primarily creating policies that are expected to protect and promote trust. This has implications for government communication about immunization and, more specifically, for how to respond to vaccine misinformation in the public arena.

9.2   "Building and Maintaining" Trust in Vaccination?

It is vital that immunization programs are generally endorsed by the public and that a large majority of citizens are intrinsically motivated to participate. Successful collective protection against infectious diseases is not only determined by the effectiveness of vaccines provided but also by the level and depth of trust citizens have in vaccinations, medical staff, and public health institutions. This suggests that governments should invest a great deal of energy in public trust in voluntary vaccination, which also requires that government actively encourages those who are still hesitant to get on board. Governments indeed have the ability to make vaccines accessible through collective programs and promote acceptance through communication and information programs. As Attwell et al. (2022) state, "Nobody is born wanting to get vaccinated. Every generation and social group across the world must be socialized into the practice" (p. 576). Governmental agencies should do their utmost best to make the choice to vaccinate the normal choice.

Still, there remains a precarious balance between active vaccination promotion and socialization by the government and citizens' trust in vaccination. How should we understand trust in vaccination, or vaccine confidence, and how can this be promoted? The Vaccine Confidence Project, led by Heidi Larson of the London School of Hygiene and Tropical Medicine, defines vaccine confidence as "the belief that vaccination—and by extension the providers and range of private sector and political entities behind it—serves the best health interests of the public and its constituents" (Vaccine Confidence Project, 2020). But trust is more than a belief. In section 2.4, we explained that trust involves deferring with comfort and confidence to others, about something beyond one's knowledge or power, in ways that can potentially hurt oneself. This mental state has different elements: a *willingness* to defer to the judgments of other persons, a *feeling* that this willingness will not be abused, and a complex set of *beliefs* that offers (limited, not complete) support for deferring to the judgment of these others. Many different factors influence people's acceptance of vaccination programs. Being well informed is certainly not the only one. According to Larson,

> Vaccine acceptance is about a relationship, about putting trust in scientists who design and develop vaccines, industries that produce them, health professionals who deliver them, and the institutions that govern them. That trust chain is a far more important lever of acceptance than any piece of information. Without these layers of confidence, even the more scientifically proven and well-communicated information may not be trusted. (Larson, 2020, p. xxxv)

Moreover, providing good and reliable information is *sine qua non* for vaccination policies, but even that is not as straightforward as it may sound. It can be very difficult to judge what information on effectiveness and safety and which scientific uncertainties must be shared in public information campaigns—and this is particularly important for vaccine confidence. Especially in the context of new diseases and recently developed vaccines, evolving insights and epidemiological developments imply that medical experts learn on the fly. New vaccines are not allowed on the market until they have been tested on tens of thousands of persons and have been found to be safe and effective in those tests. A very rare side effect, however, will only come to

---

Box 9.1
COVID-19 Vaccines: Adverse Effects and Public Trust

In the course of the COVID-19 vaccination program, it became clear that the non-mRNA vaccines created by AstraZeneca and Johnson & Johnson had a very rare but serious thrombosis-like side effect. It seemed to occur more frequently in young people, although it turned out to be notoriously difficult to indicate the youngest age at which the side effect was potentially likely to occur. Data showed that the adverse effect occurred more frequently among young women, but this might have been caused by a confounder, because in the early stage of pandemic vaccination, nursing staff were among the first to get their shots, and this group consists mainly of women. This caused a difficult dilemma for public health authorities: how should they respond to the very small and still uncertain risk? Should governments decide to prioritize precaution and safety—almost at all costs—and stop using these vaccines, even though this decision might will cost more lives than it saved? Or should they take a more consequentialist approach during the pandemic and continue to vaccinate en masse, which would save most lives but also cause the death of some individuals due to this rare adverse effect (Pierik, 2021b)? This dilemma obviously also had an impact on how citizens—already often reluctant due to the speed of COVID-19 vaccine development—perceived safety. When it was decided in some countries that the AstraZeneca and the Johnson & Johnson vaccines would no longer be offered to younger persons, many older people wanted to receive the alternative options as well.

---

light when millions have received the vaccine. And because such a side effect is so rare, it will also take some time to find out whether it has indeed been caused by the vaccine. The evidence that this condition could indeed be a side effect of the vaccine may only slowly come to the surface through initially contradicting study reports that may not even have been peer reviewed yet. This creates a dilemma for expert advisory bodies and governments: how should they deal with uncertainty, knowing that such information will affect how the public perceive the vaccine?

So, even though providing reliable information is essential for people to be able to trust vaccination policies, it is often impossible to present a clear and univocal message, especially in response to concerns about safety. This was one of the factors that at least for some time hampered the COVID-19 mass vaccination campaign (box 9.1).

Given how essential widespread vaccine confidence is for successful protection against infectious diseases, it is understandable that public health authorities want to build and maintain public trust. However, it is not obvious that they can do so. Confidence is not something that an organization that wants to be trusted can "make" or cause to exist. The relational attitude of the "trustor" cannot be enforced or created by a "trustee." It involves an overall judgment of the trustor about the quality of the actions, policies, and actors involved in the "trustee" (i.e., the vaccination program). This judgment can be explicit and well considered or something that is just taken for granted and hardly reflected on. As Larson (2020) emphasizes, various factors influence how trust arises—or breaks down. The myriad interactions between these cognitive, emotional, socioeconomic, and cultural aspects at stake are complex, hard to understand, and difficult for governments to influence in a particular direction.

But *if* these factors were moldable to some extent, it would be questionable for institutions to actively and systematically seek to influence them with the aim of building, promoting, and sustaining public trust. Suppose that the Vaccine Confidence Project is successful in identifying and untangling the many factors that influence people's trust in vaccination. And imagine now that behavioral economists, psychologists, communication specialists, and other social scientists employed by the Department of Health developed a program that is effective in tweaking all factors in such a way that people's trust in vaccination would increase. In this hypothetical program, the government would see all information it shares about vaccination as a means to promote acceptance. All aspects of vaccine communication would be judged and shaped in a strategic way to promote a positive perception of immunization and thus strengthen confidence and take away doubts. Would it be a good idea to implement this program? The government has an important responsibility, of course, to promote vaccination and to maintain herd immunity. Yet implementing such an all-encompassing policy to influence people's trust is not unproblematic.

First, there is something disrespectful for a government to shape all information processes, communication policies, and other social factors in a manner that maximizes the public's confidence in government policy and governmental actors. Information and communication then become not elements that enable people to make their *own* judgments and decisions, on the basis of their own values, but elements that influence their perception and judgment in such a way that they will choose what the government prefers them to choose. Of course, some degree of influencing perception and judgment is part and parcel of any effective communication. As mentioned earlier in this section, governmental agencies should do their utmost best to socialize citizens into accepting vaccination and to make the choice to vaccinate the normal, or even "banal," choice (Attwell et al., 2021; Attwell et al., 2022, p. 575; Conis, 2015). But communication should not turn into manipulation.[1] If communication is fully tailored to maximize the effect, this does not fit with a respectful relationship and might backfire in the long run. The most important thing is that information is honest and well grounded, so that the trust that might be given is also justified (O'Neill, 2018). If government, public health authorities, or health professionals are concerned about public trust in vaccination—and they should be—the appropriate thing to focus on is to ensure that they are themselves trustworthy (cf. Meijboom et al., 2006; O'Neill, 2018). That is what they can and should influence. Interestingly, this is only possible if the trustee (i.e., the government) is prepared to "give trust" to citizens as well: to have confidence that, if they have the appropriate information, citizens are capable of making a good judgment about what to do. In this way, we can see trust as a *mutual relationship* between (in this case) public health authorities (or government) and citizens. Governments should aim to build, strengthen, and maintain relationships of trust, and this sets limits to how far they can go in tailoring communication processes in such a way that as many people as possible will believe that vaccines are effective and safe.

Second, without such a relationship of trust, it is also questionable whether government communication can successfully maintain vaccine confidence that is sufficiently robust to withstand the cases of adverse effects and vaccine failure that will inevitably occur. If health authorities succeed in inducing a univocally positive perception of immunization, parents may feel betrayed if a vaccine appears to be less effective or if it comes with adverse effects. As the saying goes, trust arrives on foot and leaves on horseback, and this certainly applies when such trust is based on an all-too-positive presentation of science. For that matter, it is difficult to see how public health authorities could determine the availability of information and the spread of diverging ideas about vaccinations—especially in a society in which certain groups actively spread doubts about vaccine safety. Discussions on social media play an important role in what people are willing to believe and accept. It is often not national news, information disseminated by a government authority, or a scientific consensus that is the most important source that leads people to believe something about topics on which they have no specific expertise themselves. Instead, it is stories, anecdotes, or arguments that are shared on social media. Alternative information sources can only be controlled in a minimal way. Moreover, as we argue in the next section, suppressing information that does not fit the "official view" on vaccination will not do in a democratic context.

We conclude that governments should be cautious to employ an explicit public relations approach to "build" vaccine confidence or trust, in the sense of organizing and shaping social conditions and the exchange of information in a way that induces citizens to trust and accept vaccination. Trust as a mental state or attitude of the public toward health authorities or vaccination cannot genuinely be created by those health authorities themselves. Governments, public health institutions, and health professionals should instead focus on being *trustworthy* and on building and maintaining relationships of trust with citizens.

What does this imply? Trustworthiness involves, among other things, that government agencies base their decisions concerning vaccination policies on the most reliable information available. Obviously, they should be honest and transparent in their communication, explaining how decisions came about, the grounds on which they were made, and the inherent uncertainties that are involved in such decision-making. And they should use and maintain their expertise to monitor and ensure the safety and effectiveness of immunization. Moreover, it also involves caring for relationships of trust. Trustworthy public health professionals or institutions engage with parents or other citizens; they allow and enable them to voice their hopes and concerns, and they take those concerns seriously. Governments can invest in making policies and programs less anonymous and more "human," certainly in areas where vaccination uptake is relatively low. In some European cities, participation by parents with a migrant background is far from optimal, and here a more personal approach, possibly with help from professionals and community leaders with a similar migrant background, could establish or build on existing relationships of trust. Again, however, the focus for public health professionals and authorities should be on being trustworthy, not on inducing people to trust a vaccine. Trust can be given by people; it is not something that the to-be-trusted institution should try to bring about. We have argued previously that vaccination can be seen as a collective endeavor of government, public health professionals, and citizens. This is another reason why relationships of trust are important, and arguably they are only possible if the ultimate aims, to protect the health of children and to prevent major outbreaks, are widely shared. Relationships of mutual trust are a constitutive element of successful collective vaccination programs.

Note that this argument for trustworthiness and promoting relationships of trust still leaves room for persuasive communication, with a role for nudges, incentives, positive framing of information, and employment of other means to help people overcome their vaccine hesitance. Yet liberal-democratic governments must at the same time respect democratic constraints on attempts to shape public preferences and perceptions.

9.3 Freedom of Speech in a Democratic Society

In the previous section, we argued that in a relationship of trust, public health authorities and governments should also be prepared to trust citizens' capacity to use information about vaccination in such a way that they will come to a reasonable judgment. Regarding evidence-based information about the safety and effectiveness of immunizations, public health practices that seek to establish relationships of trust, and clear policies aiming at maintaining herd immunity, one hopes that citizens, for themselves or for their children, want to participate in immunization programs. The problem, however, is that there is also other information "out there" and more forces that will influence people's view on immunization—and hence their willingness to trust public health programs.

Of course, most citizens in democratic states have confidence in regular vaccinations, and even the rapidly developed novel COVID-19 vaccines have mostly been well accepted. At the same time, a significant minority remain hesitant about collective vaccination programs, and their doubts are triggered and sustained by a small but vocal skeptical community, who actively spreads information about alleged severe side effects of vaccines or about the alleged superfluousness of public health interventions in general. There has always been public discussion about vaccine effectiveness and safety, but the past two decades have seen a reemergence of vocal antivaccination movements, which see themselves as an *alternative community of knowers* that reject the evidence that is generally accepted in vaccination science. Rather than endorsing the existing scientific consensus, these critics emphatically endorse democratized norms for allocating epistemic authority. The emergence of these movements and the advent of the internet have changed the environment around the vaccines from top-down expert-to-consumer (vertical) communication toward nonhierarchical, dialogue-based (horizontal) communication, in which some skeptics publicly voice doubts about medical consensus on the basis of their own, often web-based, research. They appeal to anecdotes and often cherry-pick scientific studies to support their views, thus creating "alternative medical truths" that have an increasing impact on public discourse (DiRusso & Stansberry, 2022).

Opposition to immunization is largely led by this small but vocal group, which usually not only rejects vaccination but also deeply distrusts both the science on which policies are founded and the democratic integrity of government in general. They are prominent on social media, publish their own books and "documentaries," and are invited to speak on television programs that often prefer to give a voice to different perspectives in polarized societal controversies.[2] Their stories easily trigger, fuel, and deepen the initial doubts, concerns, and hesitancy that many young parents experience when they have to make a decision about vaccination. This disbalance makes hesitant parents systematically overestimate the magnitude of the risks involved, causing them to doubt whether the benefits of vaccinations do outweigh their dangers (Larson et al., 2011, p. 526). It is somewhat unsettling that in democratic societies, unscientific claims, half-truths, and outright lies can have such weight in public debate, diluting the voice of evidence-based science (Kata, 2010; Venkatramana et al., 2015, p. 1422). Ultimately, these voices challenge and potentially threaten public trust in collective immunization—and thus undermine collective protection against infectious diseases. How should liberal-democratic governments respond?

To counteract these voices would be to suppress the sharing of "fake news" and "alternative truths" about the effectiveness and safety of vaccines, either by the state itself, for example, by prohibiting such expressions, or by requiring social media, internet providers, and other publishers to suppress or downplay messages, blogs, or videos that undermine vaccine confidence. In line with the argument of the previous section, we see this as a wrongheaded approach to trying to maintain trust: a government that suppresses opinions, even those that are blatantly objectionable, is not trustworthy at all. There is also a further, more fundamental ground for refraining from such an approach: to respect freedom of speech.

Freedom of speech is a quintessential right in the liberal catalogue of fundamental rights. John Stuart Mill is famous not only for his defense of the harm principle, which is pivotal to the argument in this book, but especially also for the way he links this principle to a defense of a near-absolute freedom of expression. His basic argument is that for various reasons, limiting freedom of speech usually generates more harm than any speech act itself could ever generate. For the liberal political philosopher Mill, *liberty of thought* is sacrosanct (Mill, 1991, pp. 16–17). And since the *liberty of expressing and publishing opinions* is an inherent consequence of freedom of thought, it is almost as important as liberty of thought itself. In addition to the justification of freedom of speech as an essential individual right, Mill also presents several arguments why freedom of speech is an important collective endeavor that is a necessary precondition for the collective process of finding and celebrating truth.

> The peculiar evil of silencing the expression of an opinion is, that it is robbing the human race; posterity as well as the existing generation; those who dissent from the opinion, still more than those who hold it. If the opinion is right, they are deprived of the opportunity of exchanging error for truth: if wrong, they lose, what is almost as great a benefit, the clearer perception and livelier impression of truth, produced by its collision with error. (Mill, 1991, p. 21)

Mill assumes that establishing the truth on important matters is one of the "permanent interests of man as a progressive being" and that it requires "the steady habit of correcting and completing [one's] own opinion by collating it with those of others, so far from causing doubt and hesitation in carrying it into practice, is the only stable foundation for a just reliance on it." One can only be certain that one's judgment is tenable and reasonable after one has actively "sought for objections and difficulties, instead of avoiding them, and has shut out no light which can be thrown upon the subject from any quarter" (Mill, 1991, p. 25). Moreover, even if one is fully certain about the truth of one's own opinion, it will still be necessary to allow opposing voices to enable the best possible understanding of that truth. If other voices are suppressed, then even the truth will become merely dead dogma. Mill therefore embraces an almost absolute freedom of speech and rejects an active role of government in limiting utterances, irrespective of whether they are scientifically grounded, blatant untruths, or straightforward "alternative facts."

Of course, one could argue that even if certain antivaccination voices were silenced, there is little reason to fear that scientifically grounded knowledge about vaccine safety and effectiveness would become dead dogmas. After all, in the scientific arena, these claims are systematically tested, reviewed, and adjusted if new facts come about. However, we don't think that it makes sense to separate the scientific arena, where any view can be put on the table and be tested, from an arena of societal debate (e.g., on social media), where certain perspectives would be suppressed. If laypersons or self-proclaimed experts are not allowed to voice their opinions (or are actively thwarted in their attempts to voice them) while such questions and opinions can be openly debated among scientific experts, this conflicts with the values of science as well. Scientists should also be able to discuss the results of their work for a broader public, and it would be unbalanced if others, including vaccine critics, were not allowed to raise questions or objections. It is doubtful whether such a strong separation of scientific studies and societal debate can be upheld at all. And if it could, it would be undesirable: one of the values of science is that it can contribute to public reflection and understanding, and this requires not only that the results of scientific studies are disseminated in society but also that the academic habit of asking critical questions is adopted and accepted in broader societal debates. Ironically, the emergence and spread of antivaccination perspectives that raise doubts about scientific knowledge concerning how to prevent infectious diseases is also a consequence of the influence of science within society.

The case for respecting freedom of speech is therefore very strong, also when it concerns the expression and spread of vaccine hesitancy and misinformation. The emphasis on freedom of speech on matters of public concern is at the heart of the First Amendment to the US Constitution: "Congress shall make no law . . . abridging the freedom of speech." It reflects a profound commitment to the principle that debates ought to be unconstrained, robust, and wide open. Speech concerning public affairs is more than merely the self-expression of the individual person: within the US constitutional tradition, it is seen as the essence of self-government in a democracy. This implies that freedom of speech on issues of public concern is virtually unrestricted and that government or courts should not inhibit public debates. This foundational character provides freedom of speech with a trump-card character in US constitutional discussions, disabling courts to balance it with other fundamental rights.

Freedom of speech is also well established in article 10 of the European Convention of Human Rights. Note, however, that this article comes with certain provisions that are similar to those we referred to earlier (section 3.7) in relation to article 9: all rights in the European Convention may be subject to restrictions that are necessary in a democratic society for the various fundamental interests, including the protection of health and the rights of others.[3]

This proviso raises an important question: if the spread of doubts and alternative facts about vaccination undermines herd immunity and thus public health, should that not be a ground for restricting freedom of expression after all? It may be difficult if not impossible to show that specific expressions of opinion are undermining vaccine confidence, but it is plausible to hold that jointly, the messages, blogs, documentaries, and videos of antivaccination groups do have a harmful impact on public health. They certainly undermine the collective endeavor to maintain group-level protection. This constitutes a form of collective harm that is similar to and arguably more powerful than the collective harm of vaccine refusal we explored in section 4.3.3. If that is the case, should not the state impose limits on freedom of speech? Of course, one way to deal with misinformation is to publicly debunk it. Public health authorities and professionals, and maybe also social media platforms, have a responsibility to see to it that well-grounded information about immunization remains available and is not diluted by the unscientific and ungrounded claims of antivaccination groups (Venkatramana et al., 2015). It is difficult, however, to effectively persuade hesitant persons by means of (often rather abstract) scientific evidence if other perspectives are supported with anecdotes, stories, and rumors and by cherry-picking or sometimes simply misrepresenting scientific findings. If the harms of certain expressions cannot be prevented by showing how those ideas are flawed and dangerous, shouldn't those messages, for example on social media, somehow be restricted?

One possible step that social media companies themselves can take, and have also done, is to downplay messages that can be seen as harmful misinformation. This does not make messages invisible, and no one is restricted in their freedom of expression, but it does affect how prominent these messages appear in people's timelines. And *if* social media can do this according to their own misinformation policies and the terms their clients have agreed to, there is no reason why professionals or government officials should refrain from pointing these social media to certain potentially harmful messages, and asking them to consider downplaying these in the timelines of users (Verweij & Pierik, 2023). In our view, a trustworthy government should be reluctant to intervene in social media discussions in such a way, but can do so as a last resort, if the strategy is made public and if social media organizations can and do make their own choices about whether they act in line with such requests.

A step further, however, would be that a government *required* social media to downplay harmful misinformation about vaccination. That would amount to a suppression of freedom of speech, or, in other words, to censorship. Can this be justified at all? Taking all the elements of the preceding discussion into account, there is insufficient basis for censoring or suppressing the spread of antivaccination beliefs, *even if they are expected to cause harm*. It would be both unfeasible and undesirable to really suppress the exchange of certain opinions about immunization in societal debates while simultaneously promoting and protecting open discussion in the scientific arena. Moreover, in line with our argument in the previous section, this is not how a trustworthy government can respond to critical perspectives. If the state actively censors some people's questioning of the evidence for a specific policy, it destroys everyone's ground for trusting the policy. This argument does not solve the problem of vaccine misinformation; it only closes the option to suppress misguided beliefs about vaccination. Vaccine refusal and hesitancy are here to stay, and in an open society, they will inevitably spread and "infect" young parents. It goes without saying that public health authorities, scientific experts, health professionals, and journalists have a responsibility to expose and refute misinformation, but this may, unfortunately, not be enough to persuade all people who are in doubt due to messages about alleged harms of vaccination. If, partly due to misinformation, vaccine coverage is in decline and falls below a certain threshold minimum (cf. section 7.4.4), a liberal-democratic government better implements mandatory immunization. This also constitutes a severe constraint of the freedom of citizens, but as we show in the next section, it fits much better in a trustworthy government policy.

9.4 A Trustworthy Immunization Policy

Trust in vaccination is a result of many different factors, and as we have argued, democratic states should be reluctant to try to influence it in a direct way. What governments must focus on is being trustworthy, to give citizens reasons to trust the state and the health policies it enacts. In this section, we suggest seven characteristics of a trustworthy immunization policy, thereby combining insights from the analyses in this and previous chapters.

In general, being trustworthy involves being transparent about one's position and about the grounds for choices that one makes, embracing values and goals that others have reason to endorse as well, taking the needs and perspectives of people seriously, and being competent in the skills needed to carry out what must be done to accomplish the goals at stake. Jointly, these elements facilitate relationships of trust. By applying them to the role of the state and the nature of immunization programs, we propose the following requirements for trustworthy vaccination policies.

1. Vaccination policies are transparent and based on reasonable values and scientific evidence.   The core values that guide vaccination policy should be uncontroversial. This includes the protection of the health of all (and notably of children); the protection of societal life against disruptive outbreaks that undermine, among other things, a stable economy and a well-functioning health and education system; and equitable access to vaccination for all. Empirical claims about the prevalence and impact of disease and the effectiveness and safety of vaccines that are used for policy making should be evidence based. There is no better ground for general empirical claims than science. Political decisions about the content of a program therefore require expert scientific advice in which clear and transparent criteria are applied that are based on the core values mentioned above (Gezondheidsraad, 2013; Pierik, 2021b; Verweij & Houweling, 2014).

2. The state sees to it that citizens have easy access to independent, evidence-based information about protective effects as well as adverse side effects of all vaccinations that are part of the collective program.   Ideally, every individual is able to form a well-considered judgment about immunization. Even in mandatory programs, it is important that participants are well informed about vaccination and the effects they can expect. Evidence-based information is also important as a counterweight to all less reliable information that is often easily accessible. At the same time, it is important to distinguish independent information provision from the more persuasive messages that governments will communicate to promote compliance. The state cannot and should not be neutral about people's choice for or against participation, and this creates a possible tension within trustworthy information policies. Dealing with this tension in a trustworthy way first and foremost means being explicit about it: to make it clear that the state has a responsibility to protect public health and therefore aims at participation rates that are as high as possible. On the other hand, citizens should be able to trust that this policy goal does not determine the content of information about, for example, the prevalence and severity of side effects. Arguably the best way to do that is to let an independent body (e.g., the relevant scientific advisory committee) determine or review the factual information that the state makes available to citizens.

3. Concerns of hesitant parents are taken seriously, but health authorities and professionals are also active in pointing out the flaws of misinformation or false beliefs. People who are very worried or uncertain about immunization, for example, because they have experienced adverse events or have heard stories about side effects, are not always in search of objective scientific evidence but are much more likely to be seeking an understanding, comforting response. One of the factors that may explain the "success" of antivaccination groups is that they *do* seem to offer such a response, and they do tell a story that centers on the doubts people experience. By emphasizing that everyone should do their own research on vaccination, antivaccination groups take laypersons' perspectives seriously—or so it seems. Official responses to vaccine hesitancy, on the other hand, often focus on "getting the facts right," and this unintentionally communicates that overconcerned people are ignorant or insufficiently knowledgeable about vaccination science. This may easily make them feel disrespected by the state or by "experts," which can lead to distrust (Larson, 2020, p. xxxv). Although immunization often involves massive programs that cannot be tailor-made to everyone's preferences or needs, public health institutions should have sufficient funding so that professionals can dedicate time and energy to engaging with the worries and questions that parents have. It is much easier to trust an individual physician or nurse than "the government" or an anonymous public health institution. The physician or nurse can take the time to listen, can respond to questions in a comforting way, and can tell a person honestly what they do and do not know about what can be expected of a vaccine. Such a context is probably the most fruitful basis for restoring a relationship of trust that might have been damaged by the many factors that impede vaccine confidence.

A caring and responsive attitude does not imply that public health institutions and professionals should disregard misinformation. A trustworthy institution also requires competent professionals who are honest in presenting what they *do* know and who expose misguided beliefs to the relevant scientific evidence. At the same time, it is important for professionals to acknowledge that beliefs about vaccine safety are often embedded in a broader worldview or (quasi-)religious outlook, for example, ideas about what is "natural" and "unnatural." If someone believes that vaccines are not healthy because they are unnatural, it will not help to repeat that science shows they are safe; it may be more sensible to discuss how embracing vaccination might also be consistent with living one's life in harmony with nature.

4. The government is transparent about what it expects of citizens in relation to protection against infectious diseases but also about what citizens can expect from the government. A minister of health can and should call on parents to protect their children against infectious diseases and contribute to herd immunity. Even if immunization is voluntary, it is not wrong to make it clear that responsible parents who care about the health of their child—and of course all do—will opt for immunization. Moreover, everyone has a responsibility to contribute to, and not undermine, the collective protection against diseases that is beneficial to everyone. Vaccination is almost never a purely self-regarding choice: it is also a way of contributing to a public good and an act of solidarity or altruism toward other people who are more vulnerable to infection than oneself, notably children, the elderly, and those who are chronically ill. Protection against infectious diseases is a matter of joint activity, and a society can only be successful in this if it is a truly collective endeavor. The fact that it is not just the government that decides what is in the best interest of society but that the shared value of health requires a collective endeavor in which all participate—in other words, the state also *depends* on citizens who participate in immunization programs—offers a further condition for relationships of trust.

On the other hand, a trustworthy government does not just make it clear what is to be expected of citizens; it should also be transparent about what citizens can expect of the government when it comes to the protection against infectious diseases. Such protection is a core responsibility of the state, and citizens should have reason to trust that the state is taking it seriously. This task cannot just be delegated to parents, doctors, child day care centers, or schools. A trustworthy government makes it clear what steps will be taken if herd protection is threatened due to declining vaccination rates.

Trust in government is not only at stake in relation to vaccine-hesitant parents. Parents who do endorse immunization should also be confident that the health of their child, who might be too young yet to be immunized against measles, will not be threatened by the choices of others who are vaccine hesitant. Indeed, when vaccine coverage is low, this creates infection risks for young children (<1 year old) attending child day care centers. Therefore, the policy we proposed in chapter 7—a policy that specifies under what conditions a program that has been voluntary to date will implement mandatory measures—fits well with a trustworthy approach. It shows when and how the state will put more pressure on vaccine-hesitant citizens if a voluntary approach appears insufficient to maintain herd protection.

5. Vaccinations are not simply forced or imposed on citizens and their children. By emphasizing that immunization is the right choice yet enabling citizens to make their own choice and, if they really want to, to opt out, a government is inviting them to trust the program. This affirms the importance of a program that does not take away individual freedom and autonomy. And allowing people to opt out if they have very strong objections does not imply that it does not matter what they choose to do. The choice situation is not neutral: governments and public health professionals should see and present participation as the responsible choice (cf. requirement 4). Opting out can therefore have certain consequences, especially when there are risks of outbreaks if the vaccine coverage is too low. If the threat of a possible outbreak is real, governments have reason to be less tolerant of citizens who refuse to participate (cf. requirement 6).

6. Government and public health authorities are prepared for a possible situation in which vaccine coverage has become too low. This involves a law that specifies both a minimum level and a set of measures that will be implemented if coverage drops below that level (Pierik & Verweij, 2019b). Such a preparedness plan contributes to the trustworthiness of a program—both toward parents who endorse immunization but also to those who are hesitant. Parents who are concerned about possible outbreaks that might be dangerous for their child will need confirmation that the state will take precautions if the risk becomes real. By having a preparedness plan, the government is conveying that it is vigilant and will enact measures if herd protection is endangered, but it also shows that room is left for hesitant parents to opt out. At the same time, such a preparedness policy makes it clear that, if societal polarization increases, hesitant parents do not have to fear ad hoc measures that will be imposed on them. More coercive measures will only be installed when the vaccination rate falls below a predefined minimum threshold level.

7. Immunization policies are not technocratic but democratic decisions, which require public accountability. Policies need to be based on state-of-the-art science, but government and other politicians cannot hide behind science if policies are questioned. Questions about what infection risks are still acceptable, how far to go to avoid even the rarest side effects, and what level of vaccine coverage is to be considered a minimum are all normative political issues. Public accountability might involve, for example, an annual reflection on the effectiveness of the program, on the prevalence and nature of side effects, and on the sufficiency of current immunization rates. Public health institutions in many countries do publish such figures, but what is required as a matter of political accountability is that these figures are also presented and discussed by the minister of health, enabling parliament to raise questions about past and future measures.

9.5 When Public Distrust Prevails

In this chapter, we have discussed how a democratic state can respond to misinformation and alternative views about the effectiveness and safety of immunization—and how it should not. A key responsibility for the government is to be trustworthy toward citizens, including to those who have second thoughts about immunization or explicitly reject it. In a democracy, a trustworthy state hardly can suppress spread of misinformation about vaccines, even if such misinformation would undermine the efforts to maintain a sufficient level of vaccine coverage. If group-level protection against diseases like measles is threatened, vaccine mandates are better justifiable than censorship. This may raise worries about ongoing spread of misinformation. State coercion may motivate antivaccination groups to increase their efforts in spreading "news" about the dangers of vaccines and raise their voice about the illegitimacy of government policies—thereby fueling public distrust.

Now suppose that such distrust would prevail in a country that has implemented mandatory vaccination for children against measles and other diseases. Can mandatory immunization still be politically legitimate when a very large part of the population is persuaded by misinformation and convinced that vaccines are unsafe? Ultimately, this is a matter of political debate and decision-making. If vaccine distrust would have become so widespread that a parliamentary majority rejects coercive measures, mandatory vaccination loses its legitimacy—even if it is based upon robust biomedical evidence and ethical and legal justifications. This is what democracy is about.

Fortunately, it is unlikely that such a scenario would occur. As discussed before, recent cases of states and countries that adopted more coercive measures, like California, Australia, Italy, and France, did not result in a significant backlash in public support for vaccination. Moreover, such backlash is arguably less likely when governments ascertain their immunization policies are trustworthy in the sense we have discussed in this chapter.

10 Conclusion: Vaccination Policies and Their Millian Justification

A very brief summary of our analysis in this book is that we have argued for a specific approach to the regulation of immunization, on the basis of a normative framework that fits well with John Stuart Mill's liberal philosophy. Mill's harm principle is the constitutive pillar of our defense of vaccination policies, which should neither be completely voluntary nor involve straightforward enforcement of vaccination. A large part of our book consists of exploring how coercion can be applied in a proportionate way. Ideally, immunization policies should adopt a *mandatory* approach, which still offers limited room for deviant choices, but in some cases, a *compulsory* policy is preferable. The exact nature of intrusive measures will depend on a variety of relevant contextual factors.

In this concluding chapter, we offer a more extensive summary of our practical conclusions and recommendations, and we reflect on the justification of vaccination policies for young children and adults. Both are firmly embedded in a similar Millian framework but are quite distinct in nature and justification.

The last part of this chapter offers a reflection on the Millian framework itself as we have adopted it throughout the book. Especially in public health ethics, the harm principle, as formulated by Mill himself, is often criticized for being too narrow and offering insufficient ground for necessary public health interventions. We explain and endorse this critique and outline how this does not affect our analysis of the regulation of immunization.

10.1 Mandatory Childhood Immunization: A Practical Proposal

By appealing to the harm principle, we have offered a principled ground for liberty-limiting measures that maintain a sufficiently high vaccine coverage to protect the basic interests of children and to protect society against the disruptive effects of dangerous infectious diseases. At the same time, any such measures should not be disproportionate, which involves considering the nature of the measures (how?) and the content of the program (what?), but also specific choices that ensure that restrictive measures are only taken if necessary (when? until when?).

Our specific proposal, which is that it should be ensured that restrictions of liberty are proportionate and not tighter than necessary, focuses on the *how* and *when*. First, the proposal entails opting for a *mandatory* policy as a "middle ground" between voluntary and strictly compulsory approaches. In a mandatory approach, parents are not given access to certain (very) desirable but nonvital social goods if they decide to forgo vaccination of their child. Hence, parents still have the possibility of opting out without a legal consequence and, thus, of remaining a citizen in good standing with the political community. Still, such a choice may be costly for them. Second, the proposal involves legislating the policy in such a way that liberty-limiting measures only kick in when the vaccine coverage is below a certain predetermined critical threshold level. In this way, restrictive measures are not actually imposed unless they are deemed necessary and urgent.

A variety of contextual and pragmatic considerations may play a role in further determining the specific content of these elements. In our own context, the Netherlands, we have developed a proposal for government policy that involves legislation for both the threshold and the nature of coercive interventions. If vaccine uptake falls below a certain threshold, then the government should implement a requirement that all child day care centers can only accept children who are participating in the national immunization program. Such a policy would legislate a liberty-limiting measure but would only implement it if the threshold was passed. Moreover, even if the measure kicks in, parents still have the possibility of opting out of vaccination: doing so will only make it impossible for them to make use of child day care. We see a coercive measure that is linked to child day care much more appropriate and in line with the purpose of the policy than mandatory approaches such as Australia's "no-jab-no-pay" policy, which means that vaccine refusers lose child benefits. We also advise prohibiting access to childcare facilities instead of prohibiting access to school, because the latter measure also negatively affects children's basic interests. If, after several years of implementation, the day care requirement appeared insufficient to raise the vaccine uptake above the threshold, the next step could be to extend the coercive measure to primary school entry or to accessing child benefits.

If vaccine coverage is declining but not yet below the predetermined threshold, government and public health authorities must employ a variety of voluntary measures to promote vaccine uptake that, ideally, would help to prevent the introduction of coercive measures. In a way, our proposed law can be considered a voluntary nudge: it expresses the norm that vaccination is the appropriate choice and that refraining from vaccination is at best only tolerated. Especially when vaccination rates are declining and approaching the threshold, this will spur societal discussion, notably among parents, about the importance of childhood immunization. For example, the moment that the measles vaccine coverage is in danger of dropping below the critical threshold value, parents in favor of vaccination will realize that there is something at stake for them as well, because that would also pose a danger to their youngest children, who cannot yet be vaccinated. This will engage them in these debates, and this public discussion on the importance of vaccination may push hesitating parents to opt for immunization, even before liberty-limiting policies need to be implemented. Between 2017 and 2020, we observed in the Netherlands, how, after a period of decline, such debates about—the objectionability of—vaccine refusal generated an increase in vaccine uptake, sufficient to avert the necessity of introducing more liberty-limiting policies.

What should the threshold be for enacting restrictive measures? As we explained in chapter 7, deciding about a minimum level needs to be based on epidemiological evidence, but epidemiology as such cannot determine a threshold. The relevant epidemiological insights will be about the vaccine coverage that is deemed necessary for herd immunity. In this book, we have focused on measles because this virus is one of the most infectious pathogens that also causes a severe and potentially fatal disease, and hence it makes sense to argue for a minimum threshold vaccination rate that is necessary to protect against this virus. The RIVM, the Netherlands Institute for Public Health, argues that elimination of measles can be attained if 94 percent of the population is immune.[1] Hence, we would see 94 percent vaccine coverage as a reasonable proposal for such a minimum threshold. Herd protection effects will, to a certain extent, also occur below this level. On the other hand, the population average of 94 percent is less safe if there are small regions where coverage is far below that average. This illustrates the limitations of determining a clear threshold on solely an epidemiological ground and the importance of more precautionary considerations.

Ultimately, determining this threshold level is subject to political decision-making, and therefore other considerations, including more pragmatic concerns, might be relevant as well. For example, a government could choose a slightly lower threshold compared to what experts see as a minimum for the elimination of measles, especially if, at that time, vaccine coverage is on the rise so the "elimination" minimum might be attained without more coercive measures. Notwithstanding our legal and ethical justification of coercive measures, mandatory childhood immunization remains a controversial policy, and arguably it will be most feasible to get democratic support for legislation if coercive measures are made conditional on a threshold that has already been met.[2]

10.2   Coercive Policies for the Immunization of Adults

If immunization is not directed at children but at adults, the room for coercive measures is much smaller. We have argued that nonvoluntary collective immunization programs can only be considered in exceptional circumstances, notably during a widespread epidemic that disrupts societal life, or if there is a realistic threat that such an extreme outbreak could occur. During the outbreak, all kinds of (coercive) social measures will already be in place to reduce transmission of the disease, and this influences how immunization policies should be evaluated. For example, it will often make sense to allow vaccinated individuals more freedom during a lockdown—at least when the vaccine is effective in preventing infection of others (hence "harm to others"). This can be done by means of a protected access pass that allows people to engage in social activities or visit pubs, events, and so on. At the same time, there will often also be other grounds for giving people access to social activities, such as a very recent negative test or having gained immunity after infection. Such 3G policies can be considered a limited form of mandatory vaccination.

We have argued that if it is necessary to further tighten immunization policies to promote vaccine coverage, it would be wrong to make the protected access policy more restrictive through a 2G policy. The drawback of this approach is that the government would be requiring private actors (organizations, citizens) to refuse other people access to social life on a daily basis, leading to social exclusion and polarization within society. If it is essential to further increase immunization rates to prevent, mitigate, or end lockdowns, the government should emphasize its own responsibility for enforcing the policy, and then a *compulsory* approach is preferable. This would imply that vaccination refusal is made illegal (through criminal or administrative law) and that noncompliance is punishable with a periodical fine.

10.3 The Justification of Coercive Childhood and Adult Immunization

In this book, we have developed a specific proposal for regulating childhood immunization but have also shown how some (but not all) the arguments for mandatory childhood vaccination also apply to the immunization of adults, for example, during an outbreak of a novel virus. Let us summarize the central steps in the justification of using state power to "induce immunity," taking differences between the vaccination of children and that of adults into account.

Our proposal for mandatory immunization is shaped by the requirements of proportionality: a government's interference with citizens' freedom should not overshoot the mark but, instead, should be proportionate to the goal the law seeks to achieve and strike a reasonable balance between competing interests. But that does not take away from the fact that it *is* intrusive and does curtail parental autonomy and the freedom of thought, conscience, and religion.

Our justification for constraining freedom fits well in a liberal-democratic view of the role of the state. Let us combine, step by step, the arguments offered in this book. Steps (i)–(viii) are relevant to collective vaccination programs in general; steps (ix)–(x) are specific for childhood immunization programs.

(i) The harm principle: to protect each person's opportunities for well-being according to their own conception of the good life, it can be necessary and justified for the state to set limits on certain individual freedoms.

(ii) Outbreaks of contagious diseases are a serious threat to individual health and, via outbreaks and fear of infection, to public health too; they are also a serious threat to public order and an open society, which are the basic framework in which individual liberties, freedoms, and opportunities for well-being are enjoyed.

(iii) The spread of infection—and the containment of the spread of vaccine-preventable diseases—is largely determined by human behavior/individual choices and decisions.

(iv) Hence there is a principled ground for democratic states to implement liberty-limiting measures that are necessary to prevent the spread of dangerous infectious diseases but are not disproportionate restrictions on individual liberties.

This brings us to the role of immunization, particularly to immunization of children, given that many common infectious diseases are most risky for young children who have not yet developed disease-specific immunity.

(v) The most effective way to prevent (outbreaks of) infectious diseases is to maintain robust herd immunity via collective vaccination programs.

(vi) Herd immunity can only be achieved through collective effort and action: governments need to offer collective programs (free of charge), and citizens need to accept vaccination for themselves and their children.

(vii) Vaccine refusal can be considered harm to others in various ways: it implies increased risk for one's own child, and it enables a risk to directly infect vulnerable others. Most important in our analysis is that it undermines the collective endeavor to protecting society via herd immunity. Moreover, a massive outbreak can also disrupt society, and lockdown measures may need to be continued for a longer time if too many people refuse vaccination. The latter implications can be considered as constituting harm to all citizens.

(viii) Preventing these harms can be done effectively and proportionately via mandatory immunization, which strikes a middle ground between fully coercive policies (compulsory or forced immunization) and voluntary options.

(ix) In a liberal-democratic society, the state has a duty to maintain children's basic interests. This government responsibility can also overrule the right and responsibility of parents to raise their children in line with their own view of what is best: parental autonomy is of utmost importance but is not absolute.

(x)   The protection and maintenance of herd immunity via a mandatory policy is an indirect but effective and proportionate way for the state to fulfill its special obligation to protect the basic interests of children against the imprudent choice of their parents to opt out of vaccination.

Hence, the vulnerable position of children offers additional ground for mandatory childhood vaccination. This is one reason for concluding that coercive approaches are easier to justify in the case of childhood immunization than in the case of adult citizens. Another ground for such a distinction concerns the right to bodily integrity, which is often invoked against coercive vaccination policies. This right is highly relevant and clear if it is about adults who are in a position to make decisions about their own body, but less so in the case of children, who cannot observe and claim that right themselves. Someone's right to refuse medical treatment is an exceptionally strong moral and legal right because it is about their choice of determining what is done to them as embodied persons in the most basic sense: *it is their body*. On the other hand, parents deciding about medical treatment for their child are not determining what is happening to *their own* body but to that of their child. As dear as the child is to them, that child is still a different person. If parents object to a treatment that is deemed medically necessary for the child, and their objection is overruled by a court order or a law mandating vaccination, it is their views as parents that are set aside, but the bodily integrity of their child is not violated. Therefore, we consider mandatory immunization of children justified in "normal times," but coercive measures regarding the vaccination of adults as only appropriate in extreme cases, for example, as a response to an immediate threat of a dangerous outbreak.

There is a potential weakness to the central role of the harm principle in our argument, and that is that one could argue that vaccine refusal does not constitute harm to others at all in circumstances of a robust and sustained herd protection. If vaccine coverage is high enough, say 95 percent of all children, then a deviant choice made by other parents will not make much difference (at least not when those 5 percent are living tightly together in close-knit communities). We have explained that refusal can still be considered a form of harm done to the collective, but arguably, the case for coercion is less strong than in a context in which the level of herd protection is under threat. It is not uncommon, therefore, to seek additional support for coercion by appealing to the unfairness of vaccination freeriding. However, this argument of fairness ultimately fails. Vaccine refusal amounts to freeriding, but it is not unfair because the public good of herd protection supervenes on the private goods of all persons who have opted for vaccination. This means that preventing harm to others is, and will remain, at that core of our ethical argument.

10.4   A Critique and an Appraisal of the Millian Framework

John Stuart Mill's liberal philosophy, and notably his discussion in *On Liberty*, largely determines the normative framework for our argument. The harm principle is central to our justification of the coercive measures that are needed to establish and maintain herd protection. We have put forward herd protection as a common good and have argued, in line with Mill's discussion, that refraining from contributing to a collective project that is beneficial to everyone can count as harmful. There is also a second way in which the harm principle informs the analysis—namely, in the view that the state has a responsibility to overrule parental choices if these conflict with a child's basic interests. Preventing harm to others can thus be a ground to set limits on freedom of thought, conscience, and religion, as well as on parental autonomy.

The harm principle does offer a strong basis for coercive immunization policies, but it is not a sufficient justification. Again, in line with liberal thought, restrictions on freedom should be proportionate and not more intrusive than necessary. The fact that 100 percent coverage is not necessary for herd protection offers some room for tolerating vaccine refusal, and we have argued that this supports policies that refrain from coercion if herd protection is robust. Note that the political principle of toleration does not imply that we should accept that such refusal is morally justified. On the contrary, vaccine objectors can rightly be criticized as making irresponsible choices that show a lack of concern for vulnerable people and that involve an uncooperative if not egoist attitude toward collective efforts to prevent the spread of infectious diseases. Some might even deliberately act as free riders in a society where most people do the right thing. Yet in a liberal-democratic context, these moral concerns should not dictate public policy unless there is a clear case of preventing harm to others.

A final Millian strand in our analysis is the strong emphasis we put on the preservation and protection of freedom of expression, even in times when many vaccine-hesitant parents are persuaded by fake news and misrepresentation of medical science. For Mill, freedom of opinion is the most fundamental liberty that democratic states should defend. Our discussion of how governments should respond to the spread of vaccine misinformation is in line with his almost absolute defense of liberty of thought and expression. From a liberal perspective, containing freedom of speech is less acceptable than constraining parents in their choice to opt out of vaccination, even though spreading misinformation undeniably does have harmful consequences. The restrictions on parental freedom that come with mandatory vaccination can be much more tailored and minimized (and thus can be proportionate) than restrictions in policies that aim to restrict freedom to spread harmful misinformation, which have no clear boundaries. After all, even continuing to point at specific scientific uncertainties could contribute to widespread hesitancy and thus undermine herd protection.

The heavy reliance of our analysis on Mill's liberalism should also give us pause to reflect on its weaknesses. In public health ethics, this liberal approach emphasizing negative liberty is also widely criticized: many authors have pointed out the limits of Millian liberalism, as it seems to offer insufficient justification for the state protecting and promoting people's health. At the center of Mill's liberalism, of course, is a rejection of any paternalist aspirations of the government. The harm principle allows room to constrain the freedom of individuals to prevent harm to others, but any strong paternalism directed toward competent adults is rejected. This liberal philosophy has been criticized on a more fundamental level as it presupposes an all-too-strict distinction between self-regarding and other-regarding behavior, as if individuals could shape their own lives independently of others. If, on the other hand, it is acknowledged that personal autonomy can never be self-contained but has important relational dimensions as well—which are arguably most visible in family or community contexts—then this may give reasons to adjust some of the core tenets of liberalism (Jennings, 2009). Although we do see that the classical liberalism as defended by Mill faces such problems and might require adjustments that offer more room for values such as positive freedom, relational autonomy, and solidarity, these theoretical weaknesses, in our view, do not affect the analysis in this book. Also, in a broader egalitarian liberalism or even within more communitarian perspectives, our principled justification for mandatory childhood immunization would stand strong. After all, the strongest arguments for liberty-limiting policies are arguments that cherish the value of negative liberty. The critique that Mill's approach leaves too little room for more paternalist or solidarity-inspired policies is rather misplaced in the context of childhood immunization: even Mill argues that if the well-being of young children is at stake, paternalism *is* justified. The harm principle also offers a basis for holding the state responsible for securing the basic interests of children. Moreover, if we broaden our perspective and consider vaccination of adults, then it is also clear that a choice to accept or refuse vaccination cannot be understood as a purely self-regarding choice. Hence, the sensible critique that Mill overemphasizes a distinction between self-regarding and other-regarding behavior has little or no impact on the appropriateness of applying his liberalism to our main subject: the role of the state to regulate and mandate immunization. Collective immunization can be regulated in ways that do set limits on freedom of choice, but such policies can also be defended by appealing to the value of liberty itself.

Notes

Chapter 1

1. In 1978, ten months after the person with the last case of endemic smallpox recovered, the virus escaped from a Birmingham laboratory, infecting two other persons. This "last salute" of the virus—an expression used by Donald Hopkins—killed one person and drove the director of the lab, the famous smallpox researcher Henry Bedson, to suicide (Hopkins, 2002, p. 310).

2. Moreover, it might be unjustified if a government attempted to eradicate some diseases, because the (opportunity) costs of doing so are too high compared to the ultimate benefits (cf. Caplan, 2009).

3. And only when most circulating flu viruses are well matched with those used to make flu vaccines (Hannoun, 2013). However, since flu is such a prevalent disease, this vaccine saves a lot of lives annually, despite its limited efficacy (Foppa et al., 2015).

4. Our focus on collective immunization programs implies that we will not discuss vaccinations for specific groups or individuals (such as for travelers or professionals), therapeutic vaccines, or postexposure vaccination.

5. See, for example, Jonny Anomaly, who defends a public goods conception of public health that offers only very limited room for tackling the social determinants of health or diseases like obesity (Anomaly, 2011). Such conceptions have been criticized by, for instance, Justin Bernstein and Pierce Randall (2020).

6. Note that it is far from obvious that immunization is always easily accessible in Western democratic countries. In chapters 4 and 7, we argue that equitable access to vaccination is a precondition for mandatory policies.

Chapter 2

1. Libertarians might still have grounds for opposing *mandatory* vaccination. See, for example, the discussions by Bernstein (2017), Kowalik (2022), and Brennan (2018).

2. If administered at that moment, the vaccine generates the most optimal lifelong protection. Protection is less optimal when the vaccine is administered earlier.

3. For example, according to Jonny Anomaly's public goods conception of public health, public health policies should not aim at a high vaccination rate if the public good of herd immunity public is unattainable (Anomaly, 2011).

4. For a similar taxonomy, see Attwell and Navin (2019).

5. Antivaccination groups spread the wildest speculations via anecdotal evidence of "alternative medical truths," while official sites can only provide peer-reviewed information and medical specialists are handcuffed by professional standards in their attempts to counter this fearmongering. The legal problem here is that denialists are protected by the right to freedom of speech to disperse their views (cf. section 9.3). Despite this, a government should make serious attempts to ensure that the unscientific and ungrounded claims of these groups do not dilute the voice of evidence-based science too much. For an analysis, see Venkatramana et al. (2015, p. 1422).

6. This approach does not curtail the freedom of parents, although it requires them to confirm whether their child, once it has a place in the venue, has undergone the required vaccinations.

7. Such an approach is sometimes called "mandatory declination" (cf. Ribner et al., 2008).

8. The withholding of child benefits may, from a financial perspective, have similar effects to a criminal fine, as discussed next. But the impact of the latter measure is larger because once a vaccine refuser has been criminally convicted, this implies that they are no longer a member in good standing of the political community (Navin & Attwell, 2019, p. 1047).

9. In situations where parents have access to reasonable alternatives (homeschooling or applying for a nonmedical exemption for school entry), we would see this as a mandatory, not a compulsory program.

10. The problem with the "intervention ladder," however, is that it suggests that the justification of coercive public health measures is only about health and liberty (Dawson, 2016). In our view, *if* more coercive strategies are justified, it is not obvious that the smallest infringement of freedom is always to be preferred. In our discussion of the vaccination of adults in chapter 8, we will argue that in some circumstances, it is better to make vaccination refusal illegal (a compulsory policy) than to exclude unvaccinated citizens from social activities (a less restrictive, mandatory policy). See also sections 7.3 and 8.4.

Chapter 3

1. A fourth group, libertarians, do not oppose vaccination per se but governmental interference in their life in general. They argue that no one, especially not the state,

can dictate what they can do with their body—or their child's body, for that matter (Wolfe & Sharp, 2002). A good example of such an argument can be found in *Jacobson v. Massachusetts*, the earliest vaccination case to be heard by the US Supreme Court, in which the plaintiff alleged that "compulsory vaccination law is . . . hostile to the inherent right of every freeman to care for his own body and health in such way as to him seems best; and that the execution of such a law against one who objects to vaccination, for whatever reason, is nothing short of an assault upon his person" (*Jacobson v. Commonwealth of Massachusetts*, 197 US 11, 1905). Libertarians can have an impact on these antivaccination sentiments when they join forces and form coalitions with antivaccination groups. This became clear in Donald Trump's 2020 reelection campaign in which skepticism toward the danger of COVID-19 and the necessity of the COVID-19 vaccination was an ingrained element of his *Make America Great Again* political identity. In this book, we will not discuss this libertarianism critique as a separate category because libertarians do not oppose vaccination *ipso facto*.

2. In chapter 6, we discuss how much weight the liberal-democratic state should give to religious, as opposed to nonreligious, opposition to vaccination.

3. Antivaccination groups typically forgo the "*anti*vaccination" label but present themselves as ex-vaxxers: "we used to follow the herd, but now we are enlightened"— or as "critical" of vaccination, employing general names such as the International Medical Council on Vaccination and the Dutch Association for Critical Vaccination (Nederlandse Vereniging voor Kritisch Prikken), and using slogans like "Vaccination is a choice. Your choice. No duty. Enlighten yourself and find your own information."

4. It remains an open question whether the current antivaccination movement is a new phenomenon or merely a new round of an old discussion. The historian Mark Largent (2012) emphasizes that there are only very few historical links between the "current" antivaccination movement (as it stood during the first decade or so of the twenty-first century) and previous movements.

5. Research by Amin et al. (2017) shows that appeals to the collective benefits of vaccination do not seem to motivate provaccination behavior among vaccine-hesitant people.

6. For example, only 0.5 percent of Italians identify themselves as "antivaccinated" (D'Ancona et al., 2019).

7. In addition, Jonathan Herring and Jesse Wall argue that bodily integrity is an important factor in and of itself and that it cannot be reduced to autonomy alone (Herring & Wall, 2017).

8. *X and Y v. the Netherlands*, App. No. 8978/80 (ECtHR, 26 March 1985), §22.

9. *Acmanne and Others v. Belgium*, p. 255; cf. *Y.F. v. Turkey*, App. No. 24209/94 (ECtHR, 22 July 2003), §33.

10. How far the bodily sphere extends, and thus also what counts as an invasion of that sphere, is a contested issue that also depends on the judgment of the person

who has the authority to decide about what is allowed or not—think, for example, about cutting someone's hair against their will. Normally, it is of course the person whose body it is who has that authority.

11. *Campbell and Cosans v. The United Kingdom*, App. Nos. 7511/76, 7743/76, Eur. Ct. H.R., at 12–13 (1982).

Chapter 4

1. In many other parts of the world, the disease is still dominantly present. In 2019, more than 200,000 people died of measles, mostly children under the age of five (Patel et al., 2020).

2. In this chapter, we do not specify what form these liberty-limiting vaccination policies will take, for example, whether they will be mandatory or compulsory. We only make the argument that the state is, in specific circumstances, allowed to limit the individual freedom not to vaccinate. In chapters 6 and 7, we elaborate on the specific form these policies should take regarding childhood vaccination and, in chapter 8, for vaccination for adults.

3. In section 10.4, we reflect on the limitations of a Millian approach to public health ethics.

4. Much more discussion is possible about the acts-omissions distinction, on both theoretical and practical levels. Regarding the latter, childhood immunization is usually offered proactively as part of a program in which parents are urged to vaccinate their children; the vaccinations may even be considered part of the basic health care package to which every child should have access. In such a context, forgoing the offer is clearly a deliberate choice (even a decision "against the current"), and in that sense, it is not obvious at all that this is a matter of "inaction."

5. We take the fairness in "doing one's fair share" in the first place as setting upper limits on what the state can require of citizens. An individual person or small group cannot be required, as a matter of preventing harm, to bear all the costs needed for the realization of a public good, given that many if not all must contribute. Later, we also discuss whether fairness also constitutes an independent justification for compulsion, so that everyone should do *at least* their fair share.

6. A theoretical difference between the collective good of dikes and that of herd protection is that the former could, in theory, be established by one single wealthy benefactor, whereas the establishment of herd immunity requires the cooperation of many.

7. This is what Brian Barry called a public interest: an interest that every person has as a *member of the public* (Barry, 1965, p. 190ff; see also Verweij, 2000, pp. 51–67).

8. This argument might also be framed in consequentialist grounds, claiming that herd immunity is a necessary goal and that mandatory policies are the best way of

achieving this within limited time. Mill would probably not disagree, as he sees the harm principle as being consistent with his broader utilitarianism.

9. The idea of "fairly allocated" or a fair share in the collective endeavor is discussed in more depth in section 4.4.1.

10. We are grateful to Mark Navin, who helped us to develop this analogy argument.

11. *Jacobson v. Massachusetts*, 197 U.S. 11, 70 (1905); see also Albert et al. (2001).

12. *Solomakhin v. Ukraine*, App No. 24429/03 (ECtHR, 15 March 2012); *Boffa and others v. San Marino*, App No. 26536/95 (Commission Decision, 15 January 1998). See also Camilleri (2019).

13. Section 4.4 is a slightly revised version of Verweij (2022), published in *Public Health Ethics*, open access under a CC-BY 4.0 license.

14. Our brief response would be that the burdens and benefits of a public good should not be assessed from a merely subjective point of view (e.g., building on a vaccine refuser's own perception of risk) but should take into account a more impartial point of view. The claim that religious objections constitute a legitimate moral objection against (compulsory) collective vaccination also does not hold because, as argued earlier, the protection of public health constitutes a valid ground on which to restrict religious freedom.

15. A similar argument is made by Bradley and Navin (2021).

16. Bradley and Navin (2021) even argue that one cannot at the same time contribute to herd immunity and benefit from it. This somewhat stronger claim only holds in specific circumstances. Lucie White (2021) shows how the claim can't be upheld if we take subsequent benefits into account. For example, during the COVID-19 pandemic, the attainment of herd protection (if possible) could have led to earlier discontinuation of lockdown measures, which would have been to the benefit of every individual, also those who had contributed to collective protection by choosing to get vaccinated.

17. The third element, the rule of law, is less relevant in this specific discussion.

18. As we argue in chapters 7 and 8, even fundamental rights such as the right to freedom of thought, conscience, and religion and the right to integrity of the body can sometimes be overruled by a democratic majority.

Chapter 5

1. See also Archard (1993, p. 113), Chervenak et al. (2016), and Dawson (2005).

2. This terminology and argumentation are very much inspired by the distinction between best and basic interests as proposed by Shapiro (1999).

3. Since the notion "what is best for their child" can lead to conflicting claims, for example, in families with children with special needs, parents are often best situated to assess and balance the competing interests of family members. This implies that they sometimes have to make difficult choices when their children's interests conflict (Diekema, 2004, p. 244).

4. Even though there is no evidence that thimerosal is harmful, it has been removed from all childhood vaccines since 2000 to forestall parental anxiety.

5. Parents who object to vaccination for religious reasons might not dispute the mainstream medical assessment of the risks and benefits of vaccination, and they might even concede that immunization is in the medical best interest of their child. The preventive intervention is considered wrong because it reflects a lack of confidence in the will of God.

6. On the interrelationship between parental rights and parental responsibilities, see Archard (2010) and Millum (2018).

7. An additional relevant factor in the analogy using the Jehovah's Witness case is that from a medical, and possibly also a legal perspective, forced vaccination, involving only a simple and brief intervention, is also less intrusive than a forced blood transfusion.

Chapter 6

1. For an overview of the history of school-based vaccine mandates, see Conis (2015) and Colgrove (2006). While there were some school mandates in the US in the nineteenth and early twentieth centuries, it wasn't until the 1960s and 1970s that US states had really effective (and enforced!) school entry mandates.

2. Some central contributions to this debate are made by Greene (2009), Jones (2014), Mahoney (2011), Sandberg and Doe (2007), Seglow (2011), Shorten (2015), and Vallier (2016).

3. For a discussion of exemptions that do violate the rights of others and, thus, are much more contested, see Cohen (2015).

4. Although concepts like state neutrality and secular law are contested within the liberal tradition (cf. Pierik & Van der Burg, 2014), it is beyond dispute that government cannot randomly distribute exemptions from mandatory law by including some groups and excluding others without good arguments justifying this distinction.

5. Nyathi et al. (2019) showed that getting rid of vaccination exemptions in California implied that vaccination coverage rose preeminently in regions where vaccination coverage was lowest, "the outbreak hotspots," sometimes by as much as 26 percentage points.

6. For an overview, see Calandrillo (2004, pp. 386–387).

7. *Dalli v. Bd. Of Educ.*, 267 N.E.2d 219, 222–23 (Mass. 1971), as quoted in Calandrillo (2004, pp. 386–387).

8. *Brown v. Stone*, 378 So.2d 218 (Miss. 1979).

9. One interesting way to deal with this issue is Cécile Laborde's disaggregation approach (2015, pp. 593–599).

10. *United States v. Seeger*, 380 US 163 (1965, p. 176).

11. *Campbell and Cosans v. The United Kingdom*, App. Nos. 7511/76, 7743/76, Eur. Ct. H.R., at 12–13 (1982).

12. Article 9 of the ECHR protects the right of a person to manifest belief through "worship, teaching, practice and observance." A "manifestation" implies a perception on the part of the person involved that a course of action is prescribed or required (Murdoch, 2007, p. 15). Up to the time of writing, there is no case law that has settled whether the right to *hold* the belief that mandatory vaccination should be resisted also implies the right to *manifest* that belief. Although this uncharted territory is quite relevant in the discussion on exemptions from mandatory vaccination, it would affect both religious and secular claims and is therefore irrelevant for this discussion at hand.

Chapter 7

1. We take the principle of proportionality as an overall legal judgment that encompasses several criteria. André Krom, for example, argues that applying the harm principle involves taking three conditions of reasonableness into account: the measure should be effective, it should not be larger than necessary (subsidiarity), and the infringement of freedom should be proportionate to the magnitude of harm to be averted (proportionality in a narrow sense) (Krom, 2016, p. 135). Our approach includes these as different elements of the principle of proportionality.

2. *Soering v. the United Kingdom*, EctHR (7 July 1989), 14038/88, para. 89.

3. These denominations are *de Gereformeerde Gemeenten in Nederland* and the *Oud Gereformeerde Gemeenten* (Pierik, 2013; Zwemer, 2001, pp. 14–19).

4. This way of presenting the argument has many similarities to how Mark Navin and Katie Attwell (2019) structured their article.

5. For a similar discussion, see Mello et al. (2020), who argue that it was wrong to even consider COVID-19 vaccination mandates until countries had put a lot of effort into persuasion and education campaigns.

6. See Pierik and Verweij (2019b) for an in-depth critique of the bill.

7. It cannot be required that infants are already *fully* vaccinated at day care entry; the requirement should be that they get their vaccinations when these are due. This implies their vaccine status needs to be checked regularly.

8. Some argue, and some even with good arguments, that day care attendance also benefits children, because it contributes to language acquisition, the learning of social skills, and getting accustomed to the rhythm of the day. It prepares children in a play-centered way for the school rhythm to follow. But the fact that school attendance is required by law and day care attendance is optional implies that the latter is seen as less essential for children's development.

9. The more coercive a program gets, the more it makes sense for the government to also set up something like the US National Vaccine Injury Compensation Program, better known as the *Vaccine Court*. This court may give financial compensation to individuals who file a petition and are found to have been injured by a vaccine that is covered by the program. Even in cases in which such a finding is not made, petitioners may receive compensation through a settlement (Health Resources & Services Administration, 2022). The basic idea is that since vaccination programs not only benefit the individual vaccinee but are also set up to serve the public good of herd protection, if an individual vaccinee encounters side effects, then such a case should not appear before a normal court with a heavy burden of proof on the claimant. Instead, such claims should be treated in a generous and fast way. The reasoning behind this is that the program does not involve itself with causation, one of the most costly and time-consuming components of a tort action for personal injury.

10. Rotavirus is much more dangerous, and often life-threatening, for children in low-income settings than in countries with well-developed medical services.

Chapter 8

1. This is not to suggest, however, that in a liberal-democratic society, the state has no responsibility at all for people's health (see our discussion in section 1.9). What we are doing is developing our justification as far as possible according to assumptions about the state's responsibility that can be embraced from diverse political perspectives.

2. Notwithstanding the importance of debates about priority access for the most vulnerable individuals or about compulsory immunization, the most dramatic injustice of the pandemic was on a global scale: almost all people in African and other middle- and low-income countries had no access to immunization at all, even at a time when high-income countries were starting their third or fourth round of vaccinations (boosters).

3. In some countries, 1G policies were proposed that gave access to facilities only to recently tested persons, whether they were vaccinated or not.

4. In public debates, a third argument therefore surfaced that especially supported 2G policies. It was suggested that a policy that allows access to venues to people with some

(infection- or vaccine-induced) immunity against the virus could significantly reduce the incidence of severe COVID-19 disease. It thus defends the exclusion of unvaccinated persons to protect them against getting severely ill and to prevent the (aggregated) impact on an already overwhelmed health care system. However, this suggested effect of a 2G policy protecting the health care system remains quite speculative.

5. A vaccine does not need to provide full prevention of transmission of the wild-type pathogen to curb an outbreak. See section 1.7 for a discussion of the concept of sterilizing immunity.

6. This argument presupposes that the coercive lockdown measures that were already in place were legitimate. The story would be different if the initial constraints on freedom were unjustified. Take the hypothetical case in which the police imprison all persons for arbitrary reasons and only restore their liberty when they opt for vaccination. In that case, the imprisoned persons can rightly claim they are being subjected to a coercive vaccination program. It is therefore understandable that people who resist COVID-19 lockdown measures and reject them as illegitimate will also consider the policy that releases vaccinated persons from such measures coercive toward vaccine refusers. Yet *if* the compulsory quarantine measures are democratically legitimate and morally justified—and again, the harm principle can serve as a backbone of this justification—*then* a view like that is simply wrong.

7. This may appear inconsistent with our plea for mandatory childhood vaccination via access to childcare, which arguably also involves using societal organizations to enforce public health tasks. In the concluding section, 8.6, we return to this issue and argue that there are relevant differences between the contexts of both proposals.

Chapter 9

1. There is a large body of literature emerging on the complex relation between trust in government and the willingness to vaccinate, and the ways in which governments can stimulate the willingness to vaccinate, that includes Lazarus et al. (2021); McCoy (2019); Attwell et al. (2020b); Haire et al. (2018); and Attwell et al. (2021).

2. This practice is sometimes called "false balance," in which a media outlet presents an issue as being more balanced between opposing viewpoints than is supported by the evidence, presenting each side of the debate as equally credible, even when the factual evidence is stacked heavily on one side. Interestingly, provaccination movements in Australia have actively trained the media to fight false balance in their reporting (cf. Vanderslott, 2019).

3. "The exercise of these freedoms [of expression], since it carries with it duties and responsibilities, may be subject to such formalities, conditions, restrictions or penalties as are prescribed by law and are necessary in a democratic society, in the interests of national security, territorial integrity, or public safety, for the prevention

of disorder or crime, for the protection of health or morals, for the protection of the reputation or rights of others, for preventing the disclosure of information received in confidence, or for maintaining the authority and impartiality of the judiciary" (ECHR Article 10(2)).

Chapter 10

1. The RIVM made several provisos concerning this percentage. One is that such a threshold only applies to larger populations in which immunity is more or less evenly spread. If there are smaller regions with a much lower vaccine coverage, outbreaks may still occur (RIVM, 2019).

2. A threshold of 94 percent vaccine coverage rate in the Netherlands would imply that coercive measures have to be implemented right away. In 2020, 93.6 percent of all children below two years of age received their shots against measles. Given that uptake had increased somewhat in the years before, it would make sense in 2020 to set the current level as a minimum and thus avoid immediate coercive steps. As suggested at the end of chapter 7, if vaccine coverage increases further, the government may decide to slowly push up the threshold as well, until 94 percent or the WHO recommendation of 95 percent is met.

References

Acmanne and Others v. Belgium. App. No. 10435/83 256 (European Court of Human Rights, 10 December 1984).

Albert, M. R., Ostheimer, K. G., & Breman, J. G. (2001). The last smallpox epidemic in Boston and the vaccination controversy, 1901–1903. *The New England Journal of Medicine, 344*(5), 375–379. https://doi.org/10.1056/NEJM200102013440511.

Alexy, R. (2014). Constitutional rights and proportionality. *Revus, 22,* 51–65. https://doi.org/10.4000/revus.2783.

Allen, A. (2007). *Vaccine: The controversial story of medicine's greatest lifesaver.* W. W. Norton & Company.

Amin, A. B., Bednarczyk, R. A., Ray, C. E., Melchiori, K. J., Graham, J., Huntsinger, J. R., & Omer, S. B. (2017). Association of moral values with vaccine hesitancy. *Nature Human Behaviour, 1*(12), 873–880. https://doi.org/10.1038/s41562-017-0256-5.

Anomaly, J. (2011). Public health and public goods. *Public Health Ethics, 4*(3), 251–259. https://doi.org/10.1093/phe/phr027.

Archard, D. (1993). *Children: Rights and childhood.* Routledge.

Archard, D. (2010). The obligations and responsibilities of parenthood. In D. Archard & D. Benetar (Eds.), *Procreation and parenthood: The ethics of bearing and rearing children.* Clarendon, pp. 103–127.

Attwell, K., Hannah, A., & Leask, J. (2022). COVID-19: Talk of "vaccine hesitancy" lets governments off the hook. *Nature, 602,* 574–577. https://doi.org/10.1038/d41586-022-00495-8.

Attwell, K., Harper, T., Rizzi, M., Taylor, J., Casigliani, V., Quattrone, F., & Lopalco, P. (2021). Inaction, under-reaction action and incapacity: Communication breakdown in Italy's vaccination governance. *Policy Sciences, 54,* 457–445. https://doi.org/10.1007/s11077-021-09427-1.

Attwell, K., & Navin, M. C. (2019). Childhood vaccination mandates: Scope, sanctions, severity, selectivity, and salience. *Milbank Quarterly, 97*(4), 978–1014. https://doi.org/10.1111/1468-0009.12417.

Attwell, K., Navin, M. C., Lopalco, P. L., Jestin, C., Reiter, S., & Omer, S. B. (2018). Recent vaccine mandates in the United States, Europe and Australia: A comparative study. *Vaccine, 36*, 7377–7384. https://doi.org/10.1016/j.vaccine.2018.10.019.

Attwell, K., Seth, R., Beard, F., Hendry, A., & Lawrence, D. (2020a). Financial interventions to increase vaccine coverage. *Pediatrics 146*(6): e20200724. https://doi.org/10.1542/peds.2020-0724.

Attwell, K., Ward, J. K., & Tomkinson, S. (2020b). Manufacturing consent for vaccine mandates: A comparative case study of communication campaigns in France and Australia. *Frontiers in Communication, 6*, 598602. https://doi.org/10.3389/fcomm.2021.598602.

Barry, B. (1965). *Political argument*. Routledge.

Barry, B. (2001). *Culture and equality: An egalitarian critique of multiculturalism*. Harvard University Press.

Bartelme, R. R. (2020). Anthroposophic medicine: A short monograph and narrative review-foundations, essential characteristics, scientific basis, safety, effectiveness and misconceptions. *Global Advances in Health and Medicine, 9*, 1–33. https://doi.org/10.1177/2164956120973634.

Bayer, R. (2008). Stigma and the ethics of public health: Not can we but should we. *Social Science & Medicine, 67*(3), 463–472. https://doi.org/10.1016/j.socscimed.2008.03.017.

Beard, F. H., Leask, J., & McIntyre, P. B. (2017). No jab, no pay and vaccine refusal in Australia: The jury is out. *The Medical Journal of Australia, 206*(9), 381–383.

Bernstein, J. (2017). The case against libertarian arguments for compulsory vaccination. *Journal of Medical Ethics, 43*(11), 792–796. https://doi.org/10.1136/medethics-2016-103857.

Bernstein, J., & Randall, P. (2020). Against the public goods conception of public health. *Public Health Ethics, 13*(3), 225–233. https://doi.org/10.1093/phe/phaa021.

Birchley, G. (2016a). Harm is all you need? Best interests and disputes about parental decision-making. *Journal of Medical Ethics, 42*, 111–115. https://doi.org/10.1136/medethics-2015-102893.

Birchley, G. (2016b). The harm threshold and parents' obligation to benefit their children. *Journal of Medical Ethics, 42*(2), 123–126. https://doi.org/10.1136/medethics-2015-102893.

Biss, E. (2014). *On immunity: An inoculation.* Greywolf Press.

Boffa and others v. San Marino. App. No. 26536/95 (European Court of Human Rights, 15 January 1998).

Bradley, E., & Navin, M. (2021). Vaccine refusal is not free riding. *Erasmus Journal for Philosophy and Economics, 14*(1), 167–181. https://doi.org/10.23941/ejpe.v14i1.555.

Brems, E., & Lavrysen, L. (2015). 'Don't use a sledgehammer to crack a nut': Less restrictive means in the case law of the European Court of Human Rights. *Human Rights Law Review, 15*(1), 139–168. https://doi.org/10.1093/hrlr/ngu040.

Brennan, J. (2018). A libertarian case for mandatory vaccination. *Journal of Medical Ethics, 44*(1), 37–43. http://dx.doi.org/10.1136/medethics-2016-103486.

Brown, R. C. H., Savulescu, J., Williams, B., & Wilkinson, D. (2020). Passport to freedom? Immunity passports for COVID-19. *Journal of Medical Ethics, 46*(10), 652–659. http://dx.doi.org/10.1136/ medethics-2020-106814.

Brown v. Stone. 378 So. 2d 218 (Mississippi Supreme Court, 1979)

Buchanan, A. E., & Brock, D. W. (1989). *Deciding for others: The ethics of surrogate decision making.* Cambridge University Press.

Buttenheim, A. M., & Asch, D. A. (2013). Making vaccine refusal less of a free ride. *Human Vaccines & Immunotherapeutics, 9*(12), 2674–2675. https://doi.org/10.4161/hv .26676.

Byskov, M. F. (2019). Qualitative and quantitative interpretations of the least restrictive means. *Bioethics, 33*, 511–521. https://doi.org/10.1111/bioe.12548.

Calandrillo, S. P. (2004). Vanishing vaccinations: Why are so many Americans opting out of vaccinating their children? *University of Michigan Journal of Law Reform, 37*(2), 353–440.

Campbell and Cosans v. The United Kingdom. App. No. 7511/76, 7743/76. (European Court of Human Rights, 25 February 1982).

Cameron, J., Williams, B., Ragonnet, R., Marais, B., & Trauer, J. (2021). Ethics of selective restriction of liberty in a pandemic. *Journal of Medical Ethics, 47*(8), 553–562. https://doi.org/10.1136/medethics-2020-107104.

Camilleri, F. (2019). Compulsory vaccinations for children: Balancing the competing human rights at stake *Netherlands Quarterly of Human Rights, 37*(3), 245–267. https://doi.org/10.1177/092405191986.

Cao, X. (2008). Immunology in China: The past, present and future. *Nature Immunology, 9*, 339–342. https://doi.org/10.1038/ni0408-339.

Caplan, A. L. (2009). Is disease eradication ethical? *The Lancet, 373*(9682), 2192–2193. https://doi.org/10.1016/s0140-6736(09)61179-x.

Chervenak, F. A., B. McCullough, L., & L. Brent, R. (2016). Professional responsibility and early childhood vaccination. *The Journal of Pediatrics, 169*, 305–309. https://doi.org/10.1016/j.jpeds.2015.10.076.

Cohen, J. (2015). Freedom of Religion Inc.: Whose sovereignty? *Netherlands Journal of Legal Philosophy, 44*(3), 169–210. https://doi.org/10.5553/NJLP/221307132015044003002.

Colgrove, J. (2005). Science in a democracy: The contested status of vaccination in the progressive era and the 1920s. *Isis, 96*, 167–191. https://doi.org/10.1086/431531.

Colgrove, J. (2006). *State of immunity: The politics of vaccination in twentieth-century America.* University of California Press.

Colgrove, J., & Lowin, A. (2016). A tale of two states: Mississippi, West Virginia, and exemptions to compulsory school vaccination laws. *Health Affairs, 35*(2), 348–355. https://doi.org/10.1377/hlthaff.2015.1172.

Committee on the Rights of the Child. (2013). *Convention on the Rights of the Child—General Comment No. 14.*

Conis, E. (2015). *Vaccine nation: America's changing relationship with immunization.* Chicago University Press.

Conti, A., Capasso, E., Casella, C., Fedeli, P., Salzano, F. A., Policino, F., Terracciano, L., & Delbon, P. (2018). Blood transfusion in children: The refusal of Jehovah's Witness parents'. *Open Medicine, 13*, 101–104. https://doi.org/10.1515/med-2018-0016.

Cripps, E. (2011). Climate change, collective harm and legitimate coercion. *Critical Review of International Social and Political Philosophy, 14*(2), 171–193. https://doi.org/10.1080/13698230.2011.529707.

Dalli v. Board of Education. 358 Mass. 753 (Supreme Judicial Court of Massachusetts, 1971).

D'Ancona, F., D'Amario, C., Maraglino, F., Rezza, G., & Iannazzo, S. (2019). The law on compulsory vaccination in Italy: An update 2 years after the introduction. *Euro Surveillance, 24*(26):1900371. https://doi.org/10.2807/1560-7917.ES.2019.24.26.1900371.

Dane, P. (1980). Religious exemptions under the free exercise clause: A model of competing authorities. *Yale Law Journal, 90*(2), 350–376.

Daniels, N. (2001). Justice, health, and healthcare. *American Journal of Bioethics, 1*(2), 2–16. https://doi.org/10.1162/152651601300168834.

Dawson, A. (2005). The determination of the best interests in relation to childhood vaccination. *Bioethics, 19*(2), 188–205. https://doi.org/10.1111/j.1467-8519.2005.00433.x.

Dawson, A. (2007). Herd protection as a public good: Vaccination and our obligations to others. In A. Dawson & M. Verweij (Eds.), *Ethics, prevention and public health* (pp. 160–178). Oxford University Press.

Dawson, A. (2011). Vaccination ethics. In A. Dawson (Ed.), *Public health ethics* (pp. 143–153). Cambridge University Press.

Dawson, A. J. (2016). Snakes and ladders: State interventions and the place of liberty in public health policy. *Journal of Medical Ethics, 42*(8), 510–513. http://dx.doi.org /10.1136/medethics-2016-103502.

Deer, B. (2011a). How the case against the MMR vaccine was fixed. *British Medical Journal, 342*(7788), 77–82. https://doi.org/10.1136/bmj.c5347.

Deer, B. (2011b). How the vaccine crisis was meant to make money. *British Medical Journal, 342*(7789), 136–142. https://doi.org/10.1136/bmj.c5258.

Di Pietrantonj, C., Rivetti, A., Marchione, P., Debalini, M. G., & Demicheli, V. (2020). Vaccines for measles, mumps, rubella, and varicella in children. *Cochrane Database of Systematic Reviews, 4*, CD004407. https://doi.org/10.1002/14651858.CD004407.pub4.

Diekema, D. S. (2004). Parental refusals of medical treatment: The harm principle as threshold for state intervention. *Theoretical Medicine, 2*, 243–264. https://doi.org/10 .1007/s11017-004-3146-6.

DiRusso, C., & Stansberry, K. (2022). Unvaxxed: A cultural study of the online anti-vaccination movement. *Qualitative Health Research, 32*(2), 317–329. https://doi.org /10.1177/10497323211056050.

Dixon, R. (2017). The core case for weak form judicial review. *Cardozo Law Review, 38*, 2193–2232.

Dobbernack, J., & Modood, T. (Eds.). (2013). *Hard to accept new perspectives on tolerance, intolerance and respect*. Palgrave.

Donzelli, G., Palomba, G., Federigi, I., Aquino, F., Cioni, L., Verani, M., Carducci, A., & Lopalco, P. (2018). Misinformation on vaccination: A quantitative analysis of YouTube videos. *Human Vaccines & Immunotherapeutics, 14*(7), 1654–1659. https:// doi.org/10.1080/21645515.2018.1454572.

Dudley, M. Z., Halsey, N. A., Omer, S. B., Orenstein, W. A., O'Leary, S. T., Limaye, R. J., & Salmon, D. A. (2020). The state of vaccine safety science: Systematic reviews of the evidence. *Lancet Infectious Diseases, 20*(5), e80–e89. https://doi.org/10.1016 /S1473-3099(20)30130-4.

Effting, M. (2014, March 15). Zij gokten met het leven van mijn kind. *De Volkskrant.*

Evers, J., Pierik, R., & Verweij, M. (2019). De registratie van vaccinatiegegevens in de kinderopvang binnen het regime van de Algemene verordening gegevensbescherming. *Privacy & Informatie, 22*(4), 130–136. https://www.uitgeverijparis.nl/nl/reader /205722/1001436944.

Feinberg, J. (1980). The child's right to an open future. In W. Aiken & H. LaFollette (Eds.), *Whose child?* (pp. 124–153). Rowman & Littlefield.

Flaherty, D. (2011). The vaccine-autism connection: A public health crisis caused by unethical medical practices and fraudulent science. *Annals of Pharmacotherapy*, *45*(10), 1302–1304. https://doi.org/10.1345/aph.1Q318.

Flanigan, J. (2014). A defense of compulsory vaccination. *HEC Forum*, *26*, 5–25. https://doi.org/10.1007/s10730-013-9221-5.

Foppa, I. M., Cheng, P.-Y., Reynolds, S. B., Shay, D. K., Carias, C., Bresee, J. S., Kim, I. K., Gambhir, M., & Fry, A. M. (2015). Deaths averted by influenza vaccination in the U.S. during the seasons 2005/06 through 2013/14. *Vaccine*, *33*(26), 3003–3009. https://doi.org/10.1016/j.vaccine.2015.02.042.

Forst, R. (2012). Toleration. In E. N. Zalta (Ed.), *The Stanford encyclopedia of philosophy (Summer 2012 Edition)*. http://plato.stanford.edu/archives/sum2012/entries/toleration/.

Fox, J. P., Elveback, L., Scott, W., Gatewood, L., & Ackerman, E. (1971). Herd immunity: Basic concept and relevance to public health immunization practices. *American Journal of Epidemiology*, *94*(3), 179–189. https://doi.org/10.1093/oxfordjournals.aje.a121310.

Garrett, L., Mushtaque, A., Chowdhury, R., & Pablos-Méndez, A. (2009). All for universal health coverage. *Lancet*, *374*(9697), 1294–1299. https://doi.org/10.1016/S0140 -6736(09)61503-8.

Gefenaite, G., Smit, M., Nijman, H. W., Tami, A., Drijfhout, I. H., Pascal, A., Postma, M. J., Wolters, B. A., van Delden, J. J. M., Wilschut, J. C., & Hak, E. (2012). Comparatively low attendance during Human Papillomavirus catch-up vaccination among teenage girls in the Netherlands: Insights from a behavioral survey among parents. *BMC Public Health*, *12*, article no 498. https://doi.org/10.1186/1471-2458-12-498.

Gergen, J., & Petsch, B. (2020). mRNA-based vaccines and mode of action. In D. Yu & B. Petsch (Eds.), *mRNA vaccines*. Book series *Current topics in microbiology and immunology* Vol. 437. Springer, 1–30. https://doi.org/10.1007/82_2020_230.

Gezondheidsraad. (2013). *The individual, collective and public importance of vaccination*. Gezondheidsraad (Health Council of the Netherlands), publicatienr. 2013/21.

Gezondheidsraad. (2020). *Vaccinatie tegen waterpokken*. Gezondheidsraad (Health Council of the Netherlands), publicatienr. 2020/19.

Ginossar, T., Cruickshank, I. J., Zheleva, E., Sulskis, J., & Berger-Wolf, T. (2022). Cross-platform spread: Vaccine-related content, sources, and conspiracy theories in YouTube videos shared in early Twitter COVID-19 conversations. *Human Vaccines & Immunotherapeutics*, *18*(1), e2003647. https://doi.org/10.1080/21645515.2021.2003647.

Giubilini, A. (2019). *The ethics of vaccination*. Palgrave MacMillan. https://doi.org/10 .1007/978-3-030-02068-2.

Giubilini, A., Minerva, F., Schuklenk, U., & Savulescu, J. (2021). The 'ethical' COVID-19 vaccine is the one that preserves lives: Religious and moral beliefs on the COVID-19 vaccine. *Public Health Ethics*, *14*(3), 242–255. https://doi.org/10.1093/phe/phab018.

Giubilini, A., & Savulescu, J. (2019). Vaccination, risks, and freedom: The seat belt analogy. *Public Health Ethics, 12*(3), 237–249. https://doi.org/10.1093/phe/phz014.

Goldenberg, M. J. (2016). Public misunderstanding of science? Reframing the problem of vaccine hesitancy. *Perspectives on Science, 24*(5), 552–580. https://doi.org/10.1162/POSC_a_00223.

Greene, A. (2009). Three theories of religious equality . . . and of exemptions. *Texas Law Review, 87*(963), 963–1007.

Gruszczynski, L., & Wu, C. (2021). Between the high ideals and reality: Managing COVID-19 vaccine nationalism. *European Journal of Risk Regulation 12* (3), 711–719. https://doi.org/10.1017/err.2021.9.

Haire, B., Komesaroff, P., Leontini, R., & Raina MacIntyre, C. (2018, June). Raising rates of childhood vaccination: The trade-off between coercion and trust. *Journal of Bioethical Inquiry, 15*(2), 199–209. https://doi.org/10.1007/s11673-018-9841-1.

Hannoun, C. (2013). The evolving history of influenza viruses and influenza vaccines. *Expert Review of Vaccines, 12*(9), 1085–1094. https://doi.org/10.1586/14760584.2013.824709.

Hausman, B. (2019). *Anti/vax: Reframing the vaccination controversy*. LR Press (Cornell University Press).

Health Resources & Services Administration. (2022). About the National Vaccine Injury Compensation Program. https://www.hrsa.gov/vaccine-compensation/about.

Herring, J., & Wall, J. (2017). The nature and significance of the right to bodily integrity. *The Cambridge Law Journal, 76*(3), 566–588. https://doi.org/10.1017/S00081973 17000605.

Hirose, I. (2023). *The ethics of pandemics. An introduction*. Routledge.

Hopkins, D. (2002). *The greatest killer: Smallpox in history*. University of Chicago Press.

Jackson, V. C. (2015). Constitutional law in an age of proportionality. *The Yale Law Journal, 124*(8), 3094–3196.

Jacobson v. Massachusetts. 197 U.S. 11 (US Supreme Court, 1905)

Jain, A., Marshall, J., Buikema, A., Bancroft, T., Kelly, J. P., & Newschaffer, C. J. (2015). Autism occurrence by MMR vaccine status among US children with older siblings with and without autism. *Journal of the American Medical Association, 313*(15), 1534–1540. https://doi.org/10.1001/jama.2015.3077.

Jalabi, R. (2015, April 17). California declares Disneyland measles outbreak over as vaccine fight rages on. *The Guardian*.

Jennings, B. (2009). Public health and liberty: Beyond the Millian paradigm. *Public Health Ethics, 2*(2), 123–134. https://doi.org/10.1093/phe/php009.

Jolley, D., & Douglas, K. M. (2014). The effects of anti-vaccine conspiracy theories on vaccination intentions. *PLoS ONE, 9*(2), e89177. https://doi.org/10.1371/journal .pone.0089177.

Jones, D., & Helmreich, S. (2020). A history of herd immunity. *The Lancet, 396*(10254), 810–811. https://doi.org/10.1016/S0140-6736(20)31924-3.

Jones, P. (2014). Accommodating religion and shifting burdens. *Criminal Law and Philosophy, 10*(3), 515–536.

Kagan, S. (2011). Do I make a difference? *Philosophy & Public Affairs, 39*(2), 105–141.

Kata, A. (2010). A postmodern Pandora's box: Anti-vaccination misinformation on the internet. *Vaccine, 28*, 1709–1716.

Katz, A. L., Webb, S. A., & Committee on Bioethics. (2016). Informed consent in decision-making in pediatric practice. *Pediatrics, 138*(2), e20161485. https://doi.org /10.1542/peds.2016-1485.

Katz, I. T., Weintraub, R., Bekker, L. G., & Brandt, A. M. (2021). From vaccine nationalism to vaccine equity. Finding a path forward. *The New England Journal of Medicine, 384*(14), 1281–1283.

Klatt, M., & Meister, M. (2012). *The constitutional structure of proportionality.* Oxford University Press.

Klosko, G. (1992). *The principle of fairness and political obligation.* Rowman & Littlefield.

Koerth-Baker, M. (2016). Values and vaccines. *Aeon.* https://aeon.co/essays/anti -vaccination-might-be-rational-but-is-it-reasonable.

Kowalik, M. (2022). Ethics of vaccine refusal. *Journal of Medical Ethics, 48*(4), 240–243. https://doi.org/10.1136/medethics-2020-107026.

Kraaijeveld, S. R. (2020). Vaccinating for whom? Distinguishing between self-protective, paternalistic, altruistic and indirect vaccination. *Public Health Ethics, 13*(2), 190–200. https://doi.org/10.1093/phe/phaa005.

Krom, A. (2016). *Not to be sneezed at: On the possibility of justifying infectious disease control by appealing to a mid-level harm principle.* Dissertation Utrecht University. https://dspace.library.uu.nl/handle/1874/288514.

Kumm, M. (2007). Institutionalizing Socratic contestation: The rationalist human rights paradigm: Legitimate authority and the point of judicial review. *European Journal of Legal Studies, 1*(2), 153–183.

Laborde, C. (2014). Equal liberty, nonestablishment and religious freedom. *Legal Theory, 20*(1), 52–77. https://doi.org/10.1017/S1352325213000141.

Laborde, C. (2015). Religion in the law: The disaggregation approach. *Law and Philosophy, 34*(6), 581–600. https://doi.org/10.1007/s10982-015-9236-y.

Laborde, C. (2017). *Liberalism's religion*. Harvard University Press.

Laprise, J.-F., Chesson, H. W., Markowitz, L. E., Drolet, M., Martin, D., Bénard, É., & Brisson, É. (2020). Effectiveness and cost-effectiveness of human papillomavirus vaccination through age 45 years in the United States. *Annals of Internal Medicine, 172*(1), 22–29. https://doi.org/10.7326/M19-1182.

Largent, M. A. (2012). *Vaccine: The debate in modern America*. Johns Hopkins University Press.

Larson, H. J. (2020). *Stuck: How vaccine rumors start—and why they don't go away*. Oxford University Press.

Larson, H. J., Cooper, L. Z., Eskola, J., Katz, S. L., & Ratzan, S. (2011). Addressing the vaccine confidence gap. *The Lancet, 378*, 526–535. https://doi.org/10.1016/S0140 -6736(11)60678-8.

Lazarus, J. V., Ratzan, S. C., Palayew, A., Gostin, L. O., Larson, H. J., Rabin, K., Kimball, S., & El-Mohandes, A. (2021). A global survey of potential acceptance of a COVID-19 vaccine. *Nature Medicine, 27*(2), 225–228. https://doi.org/10.1038/s41591-020-1124-9.

Leask, J., & Danchin, M. (2017). Imposing penalties for vaccine rejection requires strong scrutiny. *Journal of Paediatrics and Child Health, 53*(5), 439–444. https://doi .org/10.1111/jpc.13472.

Lévy-Bruhl, D., Fonteneau, L., Vaux, S., Barret, A.-S., Antona, D., Bonmarin, I., Che, D., Quelet, S., & Coignard, B. (2019). Assessment of the impact of the extension of vaccination mandates on vaccine coverage after 1 year, France. *Euro Surveillance, 24*(26), pii=1900301. https://doi.org/10.2807/1560-7917.ES.2019.24.26.1900301.

Lewin, T. (2015, January 29). Sick child's father seeks vaccination requirement. *New York Times*.

Locke, J. (1988). *Two treatises of government*. Cambridge University Press. https://doi .org/10.1017/CBO9780511810268.

Lyons, D. (1979). Liberty and harm to others. *Canadian Journal of Philosophy, 9*, 1–19. https://doi.org/10.1080/00455091.1979.10717091.

MacDonald, N. E. (2015). Vaccine hesitancy: Definition, scope and determinants. *Vaccine, 33*(34), 4161–4164. https://doi.org/10.1016/j.vaccine.2015.04.036.

Macmillan, C. (2021). *Herd immunity: Will we ever get there?* https://ym.care/5bc.

Mahoney, J. (2011). A democratic equality approach to religious exemptions. *Journal of Social Philosophy, 42*(3), 305–320. https://doi.org/10.1111/j.1467-9833.2011.01531.x.

Malm, H., & Navin, M. C. (2020a). Harming children to benefit others: A reply. *American Journal of Bioethics, 20*(12), W1–W6. https://doi.org/10.1080/15265161.2020 .1833105.

Malm, H., & Navin, M. C. (2020b). Pox parties for grannies? Chickenpox, exogenous boosting, and harmful injustices. *American Journal of Bioethics, 20*(9), 45–57. https://doi.org/10.1080/15265161.2020.1795528.

May, T., & Silverman, R. D. (2003). Clustering of exemptions as a collective action threat to herd immunity. *Vaccine, 21*, 1048–1051. https://doi.org/10.1016/S0264-410X (02)00627-8.

McCoy, C. A. (2019). Adapting coercion: How three industrialized nations manufacture vaccination compliance. *Journal of Health Politics, Policy and Law, 44*(6), 823–854. https://doi.org/10.1215/03616878-7785775.

McKenna, S. (2021, January 18). Vaccines need not completely stop COVID transmission to curb the pandemic. *Scientific American.* https://www.scientificamerican.com/article/vaccines-need-not-completely-stop-covid-transmission-to-curb-the-pandemic1/.

McNeil, D. G., Jr. (2003, January 14). Worship optional: Joining a church to avoid vaccines. *New York Times.*

Meijboom, F. L. B., Visak, T., & Brom, F. W. A. (2006). From trust to trustworthiness: Why information is not enough in the food sector. *Journal of Agricultural and Environmental Ethics volume, 19*, 427–442. https://doi.org/10.1007/s10806-006-9000-2.

Mello, M. M., Silverman, R. D., & Omer, S. B. (2020). Ensuring uptake of vaccines against SARS-CoV-2. *New England Journal of Medicine, 383*(14), 1296–1299. https://doi.org/10.1056/NEJMp2020926.

Mill, J. S. (1991). *On liberty.* Oxford University Press.

Miller, D. (2014). Majorities and minarets: Religious freedom and public space. *British Journal of Political Science, 46*(2), 437–456. https://doi.org/10.1017/S000712341 4000131.

Millum, J. (2014). The foundation of the child's right to an open future. *Journal of Social Philosophy, 45*, 522–538. https://doi.org/10.1111/josp.12076.

Millum, J. (2018). *The moral foundations of parenthood.* Oxford University Press.

Ministry of Health. (2020). *Immunisation handbook 2020.* Wellington, New Zealand: Ministry of Health. https://www.health.govt.nz.

Murdoch, J. (2007). *Freedom of thought, conscience and religion: A guide to the implementation of Article 9 of the European Convention of Human Rights.* Council of Europe Human Rights Handbooks.

Navin, M. C. (2016). *Values and vaccine refusal: Hard questions in epistemology, ethics and health care.* Routledge.

Navin, M. C. (2018). Prioritizing religion in vaccine exemption policies. In K. Vallier & M. Weber (Eds.), *Religious exemptions* (pp. 184–202). Oxford University Press.

Navin, M. C., & Attwell, K. (2019). Vaccine mandates, value pluralism, and policy diversity. *Bioethics, 33*(9), 1042–1049. https://doi.org/10.1111/bioe.12645.

Navin, M. C. & Attwell, K. (2023). *America's new vaccine wars. California and the politics of mandates.* Oxford University Press.

Navin, M. C., & Largent, M. A. (2017). Improving nonmedical vaccine exemption policies: Three case studies. *Public Health Ethics, 10*(3), 225–234. https://doi.org/10.1093/phe/phw047.

Nefsky, J. (2012). Consequentialism and the problem of collective harm: A reply to Kagan. *Philosophy & Public Affairs, 39*(4), 364–395. https://doi.org/10.1111/j.1088-4963.2012.01209.x.

Nefsky, J. (2019). Collective harm and the inefficacy problem. *Philosophy Compass, 14*(4), e12587. https://doi.org/10.1111/phc3.12587.

Nehushtan, Y. (2012). What are conscientious exemptions really about? *Oxford Journal of Law and Religion, 2*(2), 393–416. https://doi.org/10.1093/ojlr/rws045.

Nigel, G. J., De Serres, G., Farrington, P. C., & Redd, S. B. (2004). Assessment of the status of measles elimination from reported outbreaks: United States, 1997–1999. *The Journal of Infectious Diseases, 189*, S36–S42. https://doi.org/10.1086/377695.

Nozick, R. (1974). *Anarchy, state and utopia.* Basic Books.

Nuffield Council on Bioethics. (2007). *Public health: Ethical issues.* http://nuffield bioethics.org/wp-content/uploads/2014/07/Public-health-ethical-issues.pdf.

Nussbaum, M. (1992). Human functioning and social justice: In defense of Aristotelian essentialism. *Political Theory, 20*(2), 202–246. https://doi.org/10.1177/009059179 2020002002.

Nyathi, S., Karpel, H. C., Sainani, K. L., Maldonado, Y., Hotez, P. J., Bendavid, E., & Lo, N. C. (2019). The 2016 California policy to eliminate nonmedical vaccine exemptions and changes in vaccine coverage: An empirical policy analysis. *PLoS Medicine, 16*(12), e1002994. https://doi.org/10.1371/journal.pmed.1002994.

NYC Health Department. (2019, April 9). *Measles vaccination order.* New York City Department of Health and Mental Hygiene. https://www1.nyc.gov/assets/doh/downloads/pdf/press/2019/emergency-orders-measles.

Nyhan, B., Reifler, J., Richey, S., & Freed, G. L. (2014). Effective messages in vaccine promotion: A randomized trial. *Pediatrics, 133*(4), e835–842. https://doi.org/10.1542/peds.2013-2365.

O'Neill, O. (2018). Linking trust to trustworthiness. *International Journal of Philosophical Studies, 26*(2), 293–300. https://doi.org/10.1080/09672559.2018.1454637.

Onishi, N. (2022, January 6). In vulgar language, Macron vows to limit access of unvaccinated. *The New York Times.*

Opel, D. J., & Omer, S. B. (2015). Measles, mandates, and making vaccination the default option. *JAMA Pediatrics, 169*(4), 303–304. doi.org10.1001/jamapediatrics.2015 .0291.

Orenstein, W. A., Strebel, P. M., & Hinman, A. R. (2007). Building an immunity fence against measles. *The Journal of Infectious Diseases, 196*(10), 1433–1435. https:// doi.org/10.1086/522868.

Oxford Vaccine Group. (2015). *Measles; key disease facts.* http://vk.ovg.ox.ac.uk /measles.

Patel, M. K., Goodson, J. L., Alexander, J. P., Jr., Kretsinger, K., Sodha, S. V., Steulet, C., Gacic-Dobo, M., Rota, P. A., McFarland, J., Menning, L., Mulders, M. N., & Crowcroft, N. S. (2020). Progress toward regional Measles elimination—worldwide, 2000–2019. *Morbidity and Mortality Weekly Report (MMWR), 69*, 1700–1705. https://doi.org/10 .15585/mmwr.mm6945a6.

Pierik, R. (2013). Dan toch maar een vaccinatieplicht? *Nederlands Juristenblad, 88*(40), 2798–2807.

Pierik, R. (2015). Religion ain't sacrosanct. How to fight obsolete accounts of religious freedom. *Netherlands Journal of Legal Philosophy, 44*(3), 252–263. https://doi.org /10.5553/NJLP/221307132015044003007.

Pierik, R. (2017). On religious and secular exemptions. A case study of childhood vaccination waivers. *Ethnicities, 17*(2), 220–241. https://doi.org/10.1177/14687968 17692629.

Pierik, R. (2018). Mandatory vaccination: An unqualified defence. *The Journal of Applied Philosophy, 35*(2), 381–398. https://doi.org/10.1111/japp.12215.

Pierik, R. (2020a). Introducing routine varicella vaccination? Not so fast! *American Journal of Bioethics, 20*(9), 65–67. https://doi.org/10.1080/15265161.2020.1795544.

Pierik, R. (2020b, June 22). Selectie voor de ic is beter dan loten. *NRC-Handelsblad.*

Pierik, R. (2021a, October 19). Individuele keuzen leiden tot maatschappelijke gevolgen. *NRC-Handelsblad.*

Pierik, R. (2021b). Prudentie of zwabberbeleid? *Medisch Contact.* https://www .medischcontact.nl/nieuws/laatste-nieuws/artikel/-prudentie-of-zwabberbeleid.htm.

Pierik, R., & Bonten, M. (2021, September 19). Coronapas is gerechtvaardigd, Het zijn vooral de ongevaccineerden die elkaar besmetten. *NRC-Handelsblad.*

Pierik, R., & Van der Burg, W. (2014). What is neutrality? *Ratio Juris, 27*(4), 513–532. https://doi.org/10.1111/raju.12057.

Pierik, R. & Verhulp, E. (2002) Kan de wetgever de werknemers een vaccinatieplicht opleggen? *Tijdschrift voor Ontslagrecht 6*(1), 5–10. https://doi.org/0.5553/TvO /254253152022006001002.

Pierik, R., & Verweij, M. (2018, October 12). Wetsvoorstel vaccinatie spant het paard achter de wagen. *Trouw.*

Pierik, R., & Verweij, M. (2019a, April 15). Mazelen op de kinderopvang: voorkom noodmaatregelen maar kies niet voor schijnveiligheid. *De Volkskrant.*

Pierik, R., & Verweij, M. (2019b). Vaccinatie op de kinderopvang. Een wetsvoorstel dat tekort schiet, en een alternatief. *Nederlands Juristenblad, 94*(21/1199), 1526–1532.

Pierik, R., & Verweij, M. (2020a, July 14). Beloon corona-vaccinatie met meer vrijheden. *NRC-Handelsblad.*

Pierik, R., & Verweij, M. (2020b, November 18). Vaccineren hóéft niet, maar dan niet piepen over minder vrijheid. *De Volkskrant.*

Pierik, R., & Verweij, M. F. (2022). Over de beperkte rol van het recht op integriteit van het lichaam in de regulering van kindervaccinaties. *Tijdschrift voor Recht en Religie, 14*(2), 159–176. https://doi.org/10.7590/ntkr_2022_010.

Pierik, R., & Werner, W. (Eds.). (2010). *Cosmopolitanism in context: Perspectives from international law & political theory.* Cambridge University Press.

Plotkin, S. (2014). History of vaccination. *Proceedings of the National Academy of Sciences United States of America, 111*(34), 12283–12287.

Polkamp, A. G. (2019). Individual contributions to collective harm: How important is causation? *Ethics & Global Politics, 12*(1), 52–60. https://doi.org/10.1080/16544951 .2019.1565605.

Prince v. Massachusetts. 321 U.S. 158 (US Supreme Court, 1944).

Rawls, J. (1958). Justice as fairness. *The Philosophical Review, 67*(2), 164–194.

Rawls, J. (1971). *A theory of justice.* Oxford University Press.

Rawls, J. (1980). Kantian constructivism in moral theory. *Journal of Philosophy, 77*(9), 515–572.

Rawls, J. (1999). *A theory of justice* (Rev. ed.). Oxford University Press. (Original work published 1971)

Reiss, D. R. (2014). Thou shalt not take the name of the Lord Thy God in vain: Use and abuse of religious exemptions from school immunization requirements. *Hastings Law Journal, 65*(95), 1551–1602.

Reiss, D. R. (2015). Herd immunity and immunization policy: The importance of accuracy. *Oregon Law Review, 94*(1), 1–21. http://hdl.handle.net/1794/19574.

Ribner, B., Hall, C., Steinberg, J., Bornstein, W., Chakkalakal, R., Emamifar, A., Eichel, I., Lee, P. C., Castellano, P. Z., & Grossman, G. (2008). Use of a mandatory declination form in a program for influenza vaccination of healthcare workers. *Infection Control & Hospital Epidemiology, 29*(4), 302–308. https://doi.org/10.1086/529586.

Richwine, C. J., & Avi Dor, A. M. (2019). *Stricter immunization laws improve coverage? Evidence from the repeal of non-medical exemptions for school mandated vaccines* (25847). NBER. http://www.nber.org/papers/w25847.

Rivers, J. (2014). The presumption of proportionality. *Modern Law Review, 77*(3), 409–433. https://doi.org/10.1111/1468-2230.12072.

RIVM. (2019, September 25). *Een ondergrens voor de vaccinatiegraad in Nederland.* Rijksinstituut voor Volksgezondheid en Milieu.

Roth, Ph. (2010). *Nemesis.* Houghton Mifflin Harcourt.

Rubenstein Reiss, D., & Weithorn, L. A. (2015). Responding to the childhood vaccination crisis: Legal frameworks and tools in the context of parental vaccine refusal. *Buffalo Law Review, 63*, 881–980. https://digitalcommons.law.buffalo.edu /buffalolawreview/vol63/iss4/4.

Ruijs, W. L. M. (2012). *Acceptance of vaccination among orthodox protestants in the Netherlands.* Radboud Universiteit Nijmegen.

Safi, H., Wheeler, J. G., Reeve, G. R., Ochoa, E., Romero, J. R., Hopkins, R., Ryan, K. W., & Jacobs, R. F. (2012). Vaccine policy and Arkansas childhood immunization exemptions: A multi-year review. *American Journal of Preventive Medicine, 42*(6), 602–605. https://doi.org/10.1016/j.amepre.2012.02.022.

Sandberg, R., & Doe, N. (2007). Religious exemptions in discrimination law. *The Cambridge Law Journal, 66*(2), 302–312. https://www.jstor.org/stable/4500906.

Schwartzman, M. (2012). What if religion is not special? *The University of Chicago Law Review, 79*, 1351–1427. https://chicagounbound.uchicago.edu/uclrev/vol79/iss4/3.

Sears, R. (2007). *The vaccine book: Making the right decision for your child.* Little, Brown and Company.

Sears, R. (2011). *The vaccine book: Making the right decision for your child* (2nd edition). Little, Brown Spark.

Seglow, J. (2011). Theories of religious exemptions. In G. Calder & E. Ceva (Eds.), *Diversity in Europe: Dilemmas of differential treatment in theory and practice* (pp. 52–64). Routledge.

Shapiro, I. (1999). *Democratic justice.* Yale University Press.

Shorten, A. (2015). Are there rights to institutional exemptions? *Journal of Social Philosophy, 46*(2), 242–263. https://doi.org/10.1111/josp.12093.

Simmons, J. (1979). The principle of fair play. *Philosophy & Public Affairs, 8*(4), 307–337.

Soering v. the United Kingdom. App. No. 4038/88 (European Court of Human Rights, 7 July 1989)

Sorrell, T. (2007). Parental choice and expert knowledge in the debate on MMR and autism. In A. Dawson & M. Verweij (Eds.), *Ethics, prevention, and public health* (pp. 95–110). Oxford University Press.

Solomakhin v. Ukraine. App. No. 24429/03, (European Court of Human Rights, 15 March 2012)

Spinner-Halev, J. (2005). Hinduism, Christianity, and liberal religious toleration. *Political Theory, 33*(1), 28–57. https://www.jstor.org/stable/30038394.

Stone, P. (2011). *The luck of the draw: The role of lotteries in decision making.* Oxford University Press.

Strebel, P. M. (2018). Measles vaccines. In S. Plotkin, W. Orenstein, P. Offit, & K. M. Edwards (Eds.), *Plotkin's vaccines* (pp. 579–618). Elsevier.

Sundaram, M. E., Guterman, L. B., & Omer, S. B. (2019). The true cost of measles outbreaks during the postelimination era. *JAMA, 321*, 1155–1156. https://doi.org/10.1001/jama.2019.1506.

Sweet, A. S., & Mathews, J. (2019). *Proportionality balancing and constitutional governance: A comparative and global approach.* Oxford University Press.

Taylor, L. E., Swerdfeger, A. L., & Eslick, G. D. (2014). Vaccines are not associated with autism: An evidence-based meta-analysis of case-control and cohort studies. *Vaccine, 32*(29), 3623–3629. https://doi.org/10.1016/j.vaccine.2014.04.085.

Toffolutti, V., McKee, M., Melegaro, A., Ricciardi, W., & Stuckler, D. (2019). Austerity, measles and mandatory vaccination: Cross-regional analysis of vaccination in Italy 2000–2014. *European Journal of Public Health, 29*(1), 123–127. https://doi.org/10.1093/eurpub/cky178.

Trigg, R. (2012). *Equality, freedom, and religion.* Oxford University Press.

United States v. Seeger. 380 U.S. 163 (US Supreme Court, 1965)

Vaccine Confidence Project. (2020). *Vaccine confidence project: Mission statement.* https://www.vaccineconfidence.org/

Vallier, K. (2016). The moral basis of religious exemptions. *Law and Philosophy, 35*(1), 1–28. https://doi.org/10.1007/s10982-015-9246-9.

van Delden, J. J. M., Ashcroft, R., Dawson, A., Marckmann, G., Upshur, R., & Verweij, M. F. (2008). The ethics of mandatory vaccination against influenza for health care workers. *Vaccine, 26*(44), 5562–5566. https://doi.org/10.1016/j.vaccine.2008.08.002.

van den Hoven, M. (2013). Why one should do one's bit: Thinking about free riding in the context of public health ethics. *Public Health Ethics, 5*(2), 154–160. https://doi .org/10.1093/phe/phs023.

van der Meiden, A. (1993). *'De Zwarte Kousen Kerken.' Bevindelijk heroverwogen portret.* Uitgeverij Ten Have.

van Lier, E. A., Oomen, P. J., Giesbers, H., Drijfhout, I. H., de Hoogh, P. A. A. M., & de Melker, H. E. (2011). *Vaccinatiegraad Rijksvaccinatieprogramma Nederland Verslagjaar 2011.* Rijksinstituut voor Volksgezondheid en Milieu, RIVM Rapport 210021014/2011.

van Lier, E. A., Oomen, P. J., Giesbers, H., van Vliet, J. A., Hament, J.-M., Drijfhout, I. H., Zonnenberg-Hoff, I. F., & de Melker, H. E. (2021). *Vaccinatiegraad en jaarverslag Rijksvaccinatieprogramma Nederland 2020.* Rijksinstituut voor Volksgezondheid en Milieu, RIVM Rapport. 2021-0011.

van Lier, E. A., Tostmann, A., Harmsen, I. A., de Melker, H. E., Hautvast, J. L., & Ruijs, W. L. (2016). Negative attitude and low intention to vaccinate universally against varicella among public health professionals and parents in the Netherlands: Two internet surveys. *BMC Infectious Diseases, 16*, 127. https://doi.org/10.1186/s12879-016-1442-1.

van Lier, E. A., van der Maas, N. A. T., & de Melker, H. E. (2019). *Varicella in the Netherlands.* Background information for the Health Council.

van Wijhe, M., McDonald, S. A., de Melker, H. E., Postma, M. J., & Wallinga, J. (2016). Effect of vaccination programmes on mortality burden among children and young adults in the Netherlands during the 20th century: A historical analysis. *Lancet Infectious Diseases, 16*, 592–598. http://www.ncbi.nlm.nih.gov/pubmed/26873665.

Vanderslott, S. (2019). Exploring the meaning of pro-vaccine activism across two countries. *Social Science & Medicine, 222*, 59–66. https://doi.org/10.1016/j.socscimed .2018.12.033.

Vavřička and Others v. The Czech Republic. App. Nos. 47621/13, 3867/14, 73094/14, 19298/15, 19306/15, 43883/15. (European Court of Human Rights, 8 April 2021).

Vaz, O. M., Ellingson, M. K., Weiss, P., Jenness, S. M., Bardají, A., Bednarczyk, R. A., & Omer, S. B. (2020). Mandatory vaccination in Europe. *Pediatrics, 145*(2), e20190620. https://doi.org/10.1542/peds.2019-0620.

Venkatapuram, S. (2011). *Health justice: An argument from the capabilities approach.* Polity Press.

Venkatramana, A., Gargb, N., & Kumarc, N. (2015). Greater freedom of speech on Web 2.0 correlates with dominance of views linking vaccines to autism. *Vaccine, 33*, 1422–1425.

Verweij, M. (2000). *Preventive medicine between obligation and aspiration.* Kluwer.

Verweij, M. (2015). How (not) to argue for the rule of rescue. Claims of individuals vs. group solidarity. In G. Cohen, N. Daniels, & N. Eyal (Eds.), *Identified versus statistical victims: An interdisciplinary perspective.* Oxford University Press, 137–149.

Verweij, M. (2022). The (un)fairness of vaccination freeriding. *Public Health Ethics, 15*(3), 233–239. https://doi.org/10.1093/phe/phac028.

Verweij, M. F., & Dawson A. J. (2004). Ethical principles for collective immunization programmes. *Vaccine 22*(3), 122–126. https://doi.org/10.1016/j.vaccine.2004.01.062.

Verweij M. F., & Dawson, A. J. (2007) The meaning of "public" in "public health." In: Dawson A. J. & Verweij M. F. (Eds.), *Ethics, prevention, and public health* (pp. 13–29. Oxford University Press.

Verweij, M., & Pierik, R. (2020, March 19). Geef jong en fit voorrang op de intensive care. *De Volkskrant.*

Verweij, M., & Pierik, R. (2021, December 3). Liever een echte vaccinatieplicht dan 2G, dat is duidelijker en eerlijker. *De Volkskrant.*

Verweij, M. & Pierik, R. (2023, May 3). Overheid moet soms interveniëren in publiek debat. *NRC-Handelsblad.*

Verweij, M., van de Vathorst, S., Schermer, M., Willems, D., & De Vries, M. (2020). Ethical advice for an intensive care triage protocol in the COVID-19 pandemic: Lessons learned from the Netherlands. *Public Health Ethics, 13*(2), 157–165. https://doi.org/10.1093/phe/phaa027.

Verweij, M. F., & Houweling, H. (2014). What is the responsibility of national government with respect to vaccination? *Vaccine, 32*, 7163–7166. https://doi.org/10.1016/j.vaccine.2014.10.008.

Wakefield, A. J., Murch, S. H., Anthony, A., Linnell, J., Casson, D. M., Malik, M., Berelowitz, M., Dhillon, A. P., Thomson, M. A., Harvey, P., Valentine, A., Davies, S. E., & Walker-Smith, J. A. (1998). Ileal-lymphoid-nodular hyperplasia, non-specific colitis, and pervasive developmental disorder in children—retracted on January 28, 2010. *The Lancet, 351*(9103), 637–641.

Waldron, J. (1987). Theoretical foundations of liberalism. *The Philosophical Quarterly, 37*(147), 127–150.

White, L. (2021). Can One Both Contribute to and Benefit from Herd Immunity? *Erasmus Journal for Philosophy and Economics, 14* (2): 157–164. https://doi.org/10.23941/ejpe.v14i2.603.

White, L., van Basshuysen, P., & Frisch, M. (2022). When Is Lockdown Justified?. *Philosophy of Medicine, 3*(1). https://doi.org/10.5195/pom.2022.85.

Williams, B. (1996). Toleration: An impossible virtue? In D. Heyd (Ed.), *Toleration: An exclusive virtue* (pp. 3–18). Princeton University Press.

Wilson, J. (2021). *Philosophy for public health and public policy: Beyond the neglectful state*. Oxford University Press.

Wolfe, C. R., Eylem, A. A., Dandignac, M., Lowe, S. R., Weber, M. L., Scudiere, L., & Reyna, V. F. (2023). Understanding the landscape of web-based medical misinformation about vaccination. *Behavior Research Methods, 55,* 348–363. https://doi.org/10.3758/s13428-022-01840-5.

Wolfe, R. M., & Sharp, L. K. (2002). Anti-vaccinationists past and present. *British Medical Journal, 325,* 430–432.

Wolley, S. (2005). Children of Jehovah's Witnesses and adolescent Jehovah's Witnesses: What are their rights? *Archives of Disease in Childhood 90,* 715–719.

World Health Organization. (2013). *Global Vaccine Action Plan 2011–2020.*

World Health Organization. (2019). *Measles fact sheet.* http://www.who.int/mediacentre/factsheets/fs286/en/.

X and Y v. the Netherlands. App. No. 8978/80 (European Court of Human Rights, 26 March, 1985).

Y.F. v. Turkey. App. No. 24209/94 (European Court of Human Rights, 22 July, 2003).

Yang, Y. T., & Debold, V. (2014). A longitudinal analysis of the effect of nonmedical exemption law and vaccine uptake on vaccine-targeted disease rates. *American Journal of Public Health, 104,* 371–377.

Zwemer, J. P. (2001). *De Bevindelijk Gereformeerden.* Uitgeverij Kok.

Index

Basic Bioethics

Arthur Caplan, editor

Books Acquired under the Editorship of Glenn McGee and Arthur Caplan

Peter A. Ubel, *Pricing Life: Why It's Time for Health Care Rationing*

Mark G. Kuczewski and Ronald Polansky, eds., *Bioethics: Ancient Themes in Contemporary Issues*

Suzanne Holland, Karen Lebacqz, and Laurie Zoloth, eds., *The Human Embryonic Stem Cell Debate: Science, Ethics, and Public Policy*

Gita Sen, Asha George, and Piroska Östlin, eds., *Engendering International Health: The Challenge of Equity*

Carolyn McLeod, *Self-Trust and Reproductive Autonomy*

Lenny Moss, *What Genes Can't Do*

Jonathan D. Moreno, ed., *In the Wake of Terror: Medicine and Morality in a Time of Crisis*

Glenn McGee, ed., *Pragmatic Bioethics, 2d edition*

Timothy F. Murphy, *Case Studies in Biomedical Research Ethics*

Mark A. Rothstein, ed., *Genetics and Life Insurance: Medical Underwriting and Social Policy*

Kenneth A. Richman, *Ethics and the Metaphysics of Medicine: Reflections on Health and Beneficence*

David Lazer, ed., *DNA and the Criminal Justice System: The Technology of Justice*

Harold W. Baillie and Timothy K. Casey, eds., *Is Human Nature Obsolete? Genetics, Bioengineering, and the Future of the Human Condition*

Robert H. Blank and Janna C. Merrick, eds., *End-of-Life Decision Making: A Cross-National Study*

Norman L. Cantor, *Making Medical Decisions for the Profoundly Mentally Disabled*

Margrit Shildrick and Roxanne Mykitiuk, eds., *Ethics of the Body: Post-Conventional Challenges*

Alfred I. Tauber, *Patient Autonomy and the Ethics of Responsibility*

David H. Brendel, *Healing Psychiatry: Bridging the Science/Humanism Divide*

Jonathan Baron, *Against Bioethics*

Michael L. Gross, *Bioethics and Armed Conflict: Moral Dilemmas of Medicine and War*

Karen F. Greif and Jon F. Merz, *Current Controversies in the Biological Sciences: Case Studies of Policy Challenges from New Technologies*

Deborah Blizzard, *Looking Within: A Sociocultural Examination of Fetoscopy*

Ronald Cole-Turner, ed., *Design and Destiny: Jewish and Christian Perspectives on Human Germline Modification*

Holly Fernandez Lynch, *Conflicts of Conscience in Health Care: An Institutional Compromise*

Mark A. Bedau and Emily C. Parke, eds., *The Ethics of Protocells: Moral and Social Implications of Creating Life in the Laboratory*

Jonathan D. Moreno and Sam Berger, eds., *Progress in Bioethics: Science, Policy, and Politics*

Eric Racine, *Pragmatic Neuroethics: Improving Understanding and Treatment of the Mind-Brain*

Martha J. Farah, ed., *Neuroethics: An Introduction with Readings*

Jeremy R. Garrett, ed., *The Ethics of Animal Research: Exploring the Controversy*

Books Acquired under the Editorship of Arthur Caplan

Sheila Jasanoff, ed., *Reframing Rights: Bioconstitutionalism in the Genetic Age*

Christine Overall, *Why Have Children? The Ethical Debate*

Yechiel Michael Barilan, *Human Dignity, Human Rights, and Responsibility: The New Language of Global Bioethics and Bio-Law*

Tom Koch, *Thieves of Virtue: When Bioethics Stole Medicine*

Timothy F. Murphy, *Ethics, Sexual Orientation, and Choices about Children*

Daniel Callahan, *In Search of the Good: A Life in Bioethics*

Robert Blank, *Intervention in the Brain: Politics, Policy, and Ethics*

Gregory E. Kaebnick and Thomas H. Murray, eds., *Synthetic Biology and Morality: Artificial Life and the Bounds of Nature*

Dominic A. Sisti, Arthur L. Caplan, and Hila Rimon-Greenspan, eds., *Applied Ethics in Mental Healthcare: An Interdisciplinary Reader*

Barbara K. Redman, *Research Misconduct Policy in Biomedicine: Beyond the Bad-Apple Approach*

Russell Blackford, *Humanity Enhanced: Genetic Choice and the Challenge for Liberal Democracies*

Nicholas Agar, *Truly Human Enhancement: A Philosophical Defense of Limits*

Bruno Perreau, *The Politics of Adoption: Gender and the Making of French Citizenship*

Carl Schneider, *The Censor's Hand: The Misregulation of Human-Subject Research*

Lydia S. Dugdale, ed., *Dying in the Twenty-First Century: Toward a New Ethical Framework for the Art of Dying Well*

John D. Lantos and Diane S. Lauderdale, *Preterm Babies, Fetal Patients, and Childbearing Choices*

Harris Wiseman, *The Myth of the Moral Brain*

Arthur L. Caplan and Jason Schwartz, eds., *Vaccine Ethics and Policy: An Introduction with Readings*

Tom Koch, *Ethics in Everyday Places: Mapping Moral Stress, Distress, and Injury*

Nicole Piemonte, *Afflicted: How Vulnerability Can Heal Medical Education and Practice*

Abigail Gosselin, *Mental Patient: Ethics from a Patient's Perspective*

Laurie Zoloth, *May We Make the World?*

Baker, Robert, *Making Modern Medical Ethics*